Lee Family
Tai Chi Chuan

李家太極拳

Written by Hiang Kwang Thè
& David Cubine

Book Design & Video Production
David Cubine
Trigram Media
www.trigrammedia.com

Photography
Dean Hill

Dean Hill Photography
www.deanhillphotography.com

Visit the above website for book photographs available for sale.

Special Thanks to Dick Gabriel
for additional video support

Thanks to Dick Gabriel, Karen Hill, Dean Hill, Jeremy Martinez, Jeannie Thè, and Linda Welch for assistance with proofreading and copy editing.

For more information, go to:
www.leefamilytaichi.com

Published by San Pao Productions

First Edition: December 2017

ISBN: 978-0-692-99771-0

Copyright © 2017 by Hiang Kwang Thè and David W. Cubine. All rights reserved. No portion of this book and video may be reproduced, stored, or transmitted in any form or by any means, electronic, mechanical, photocopying, recording or otherwise without the written permission of the publisher and authors. Where noted, photographs Copyright © Dean Hill Photography. Used by permission.

Always consult your physician before beginning any exercise program. The information in this book is not intended to diagnose any medical condition or to replace your healthcare professional. The reader should consult with their doctor in any matters relating to their health. If you experience any pain or difficulty with these exercises, stop and consult your healthcare provider.

*In memory of Audrey Robinson.
A Tai Chi Warrior*

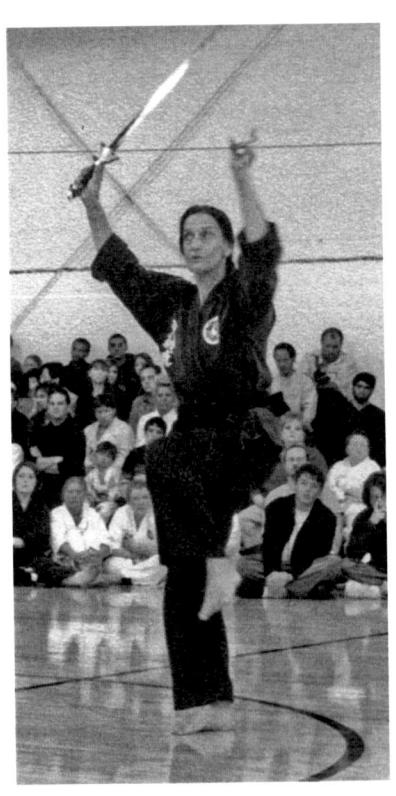

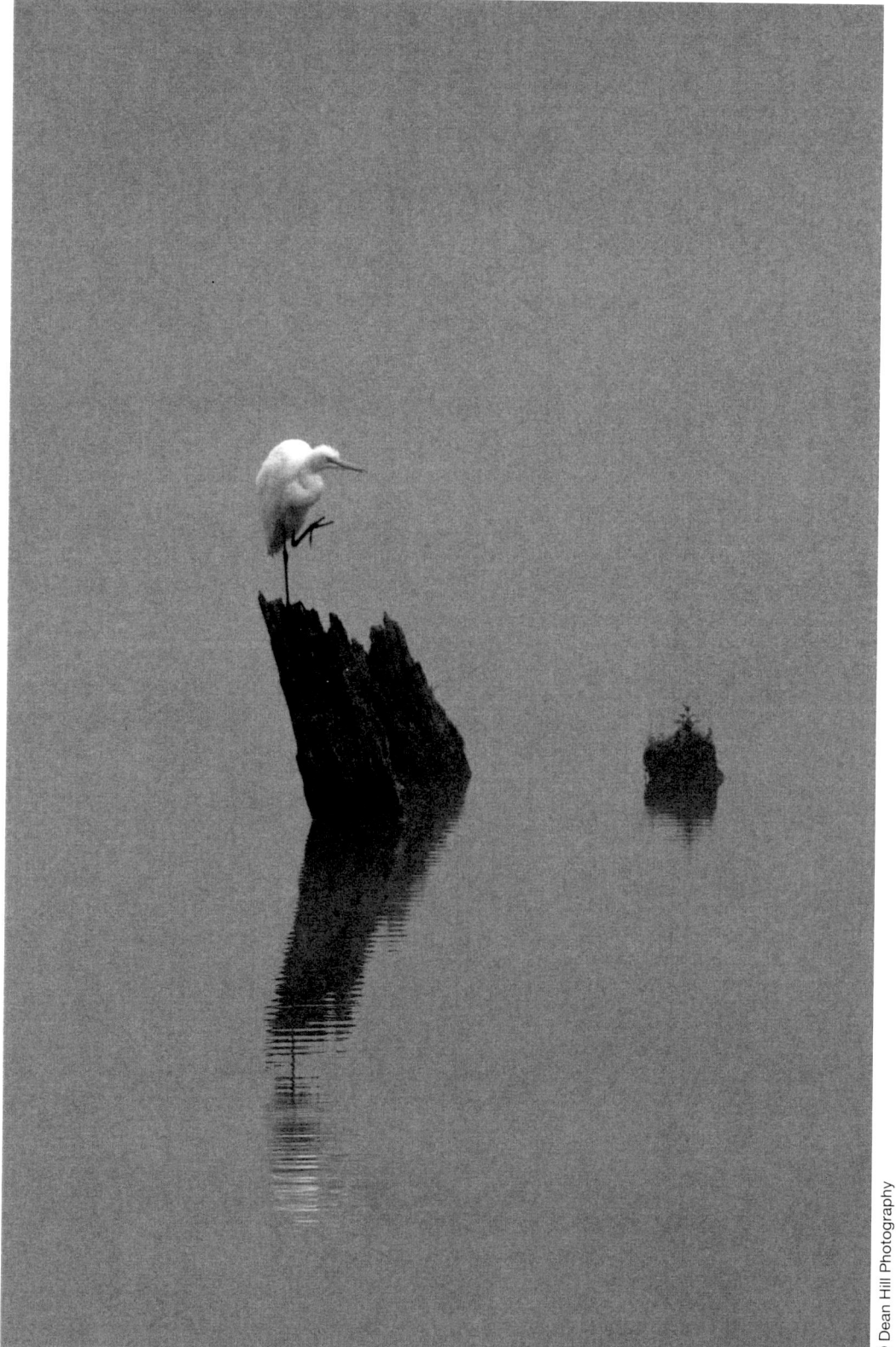

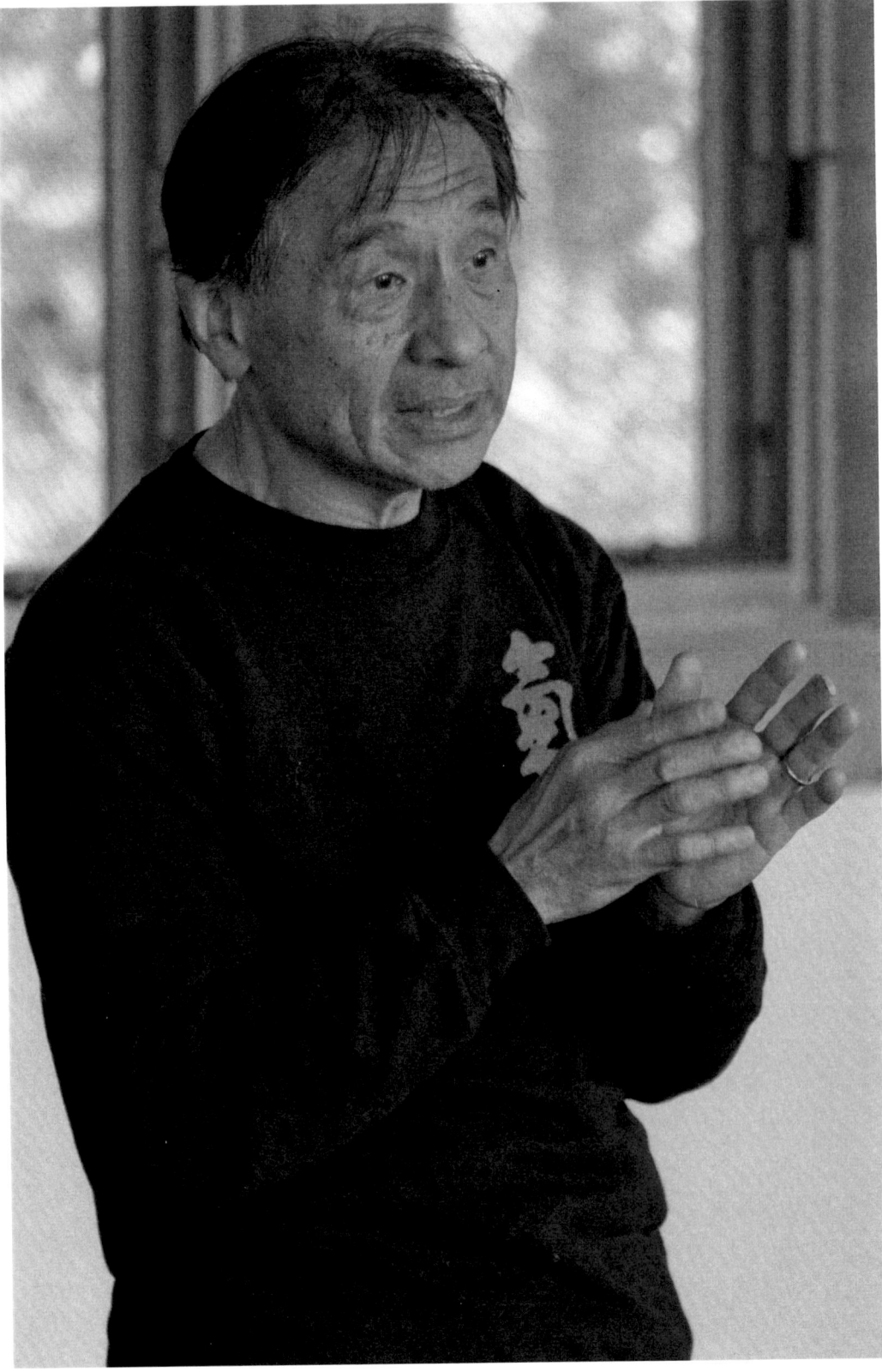

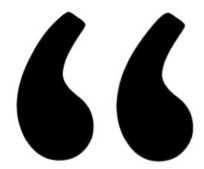

" If you invest the time to learn, you will be rewarded.

—Grandmaster Hiang Kwang Thè

"

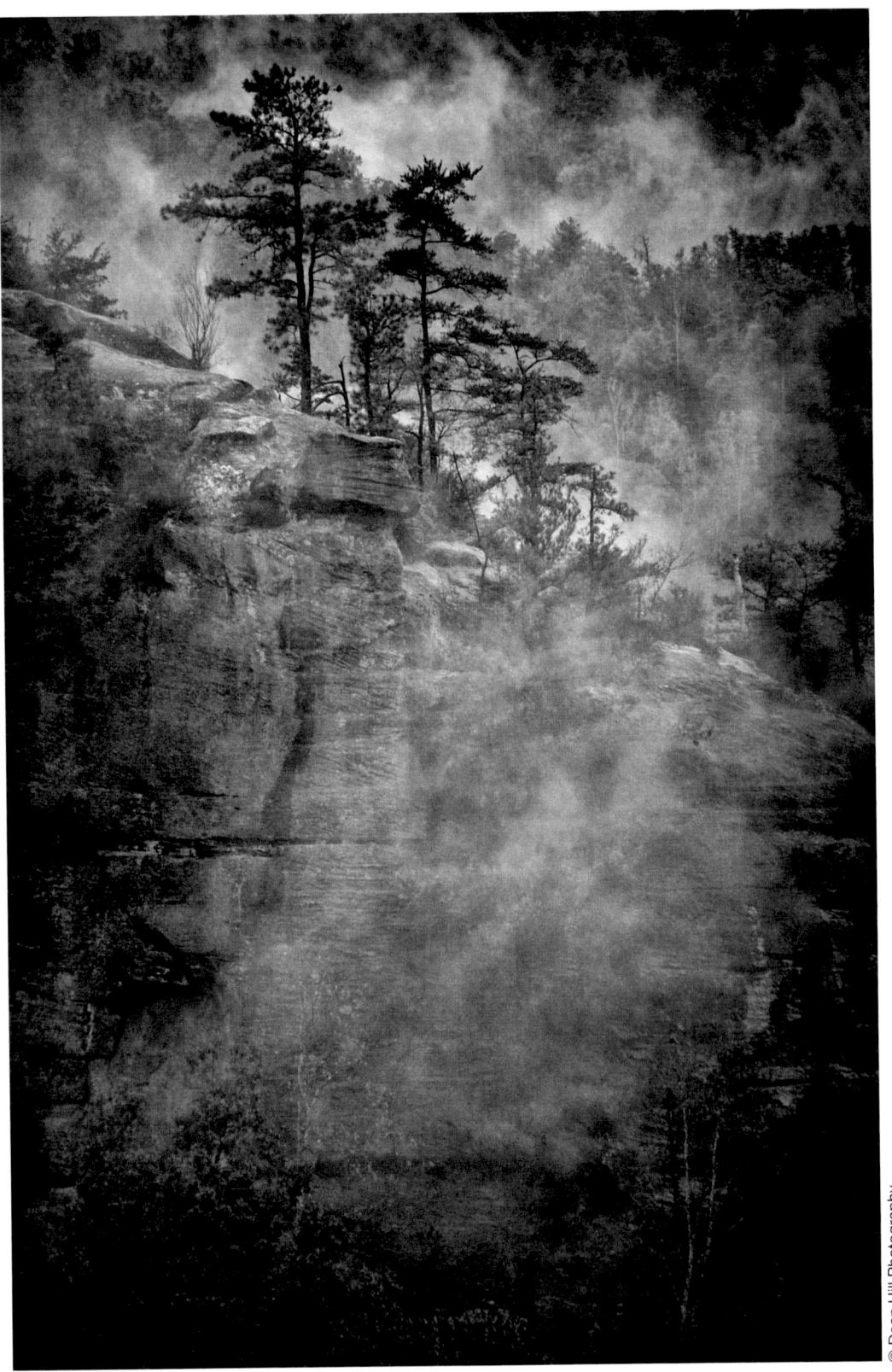

CONTENTS

FOREWORDS **Dean Hill** x**, Dick Gabriel** xii**, David Cubine** xiv

PREFACE **Hiang Kwang Thè** xviii

ONE **Introduction: What is Lee Tai Chi?** 1

TWO **How To Use This Book & Video** 7

THREE **Roots** 13

FOUR **Philosophy & Foundation** 19

FIVE **The Form** 35

SIX **Breathing** 101

SEVEN **Stances** 123

EIGHT **Weight Transfer & Equilibrium** 129

NINE **Targeting** 135

TEN **How To Practice** 145

ELEVEN **Frequently Asked Questions** 153

APPENDIX A **Vital Organs for Targeting** 161

APPENDIX B **Form Modifications** 165

FOREWORD

He moves with a purpose. His whole being, mentally and physically, is involved. Master Hiang Thè (pronounced Shung-Tay) "becomes" what he teaches.

I have known Master Hiang since 1970 when I first rolled up my too-long sleeves and pant legs of the old fashioned cotton gi (karate uniform). We "bowed in" at the beginning of class, and my life began as a student of the art of Shaolin Karate (later Central Shaolin).

Master Hiang is a firm believer in keeping yourself well-conditioned: mentally, physically, and spiritually. In younger days we went at it hard and fast, yet we were also introduced to what was to be a "new" concept to us—the "internal" arts. At first it did not make sense to me—little movement and a lot of breathing! "Just do it," says Master Hiang. I put my trust in him and did as I was guided to do…

Over 45 years later class begins with the same bowing in and Master Hiang, with the same purpose, leads the class through an advanced series of internal exercises now focusing almost entirely on our breathing and health. This is then capped off with the Lee Chia Tai Chi. "Know yourself." "Listen to your body." "Inhale to the Tan Tien level." "Exhale to …" One series of movements flows into another. One inhale followed by an equal exhale until the ending bow.

You are rejuvenated; you leave class with your mind a little sharper, your body feels cleaner.

Whatever it is, Master Hiang tells us, it's "abstract." There are no "real" numbers that show the improvement. Just go by what you "feel inside." You will find that your health improves, your balance improves, your stamina improves, and overall breathing will be deeper and more complete. I do the internal exercises including Lee Tai Chi almost daily. I believe in it!

—*Master Dean Hill, 2017*

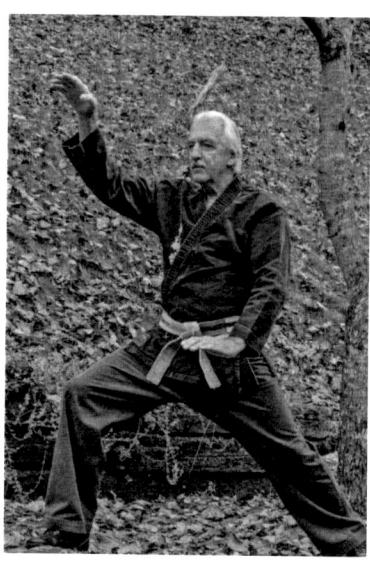

FOREWORD

There's something comforting about the yin-yang symbol. It serves as a reminder that seemingly contradictory forces can be interconnected, providing balance in whatever universe they reside. I think about that a lot when I think about Tai Chi.

We (his students) first learned the Lee Family form from Master Hiang The' in the early '80s and ever since, it has served us a number of ways. Practiced at home, it's a wonderful way to step away from the pressures of everyday life—a buffer of serenity, if you will.

As you'll learn in this book, so many of the moves are mirrored throughout the form: executed first to the right side and, later, to the left. As you practice, you'll find that while the form certainly can help you relax, with proper breathing technique you can feel it align the energy in your body, strengthening your sense of inner balance.

The Lee Family Tai Chi form has become an integral element in our martial arts training through the years. We routinely wrap up our workout sessions with Tai Chi: no matter how long we've been going, whether a grueling conditioning class or a couple of hours spent sharpening our mental and "internal" skills, Tai Chi is the perfect complement.

As practitioners of the Lee Family form, we all perform the same moves and yet, we all look different as we execute the routine. That's because your time spent doing Tai Chi is strictly yours; you get out of it what you put into it and the moves, as you yourself perform them, naturally belong to you.

As we learned Lee Chia Tai Chi Chuan, it was easy to see how much it meant to Master Hiang. He's always been a phenomenal instructor when it comes to martial arts; his devotion to and belief in Tai Chi, whether for martial arts students or folks who simply want to learn the form, is readily apparent.

Through the years we martial arts students have learned dozens of different forms within the Chung Yen Shaolin system; the one constant has been Lee Family Tai Chi. Like an old friend, it's always there and we constantly re-acquaint ourselves with it.

And, like an old friend, it never lets us down. Use this book and the accompanying video and take the time to learn Lee Family Tai Chi. You'll see what I mean.

—*Master Dick Gabriel, 2017*

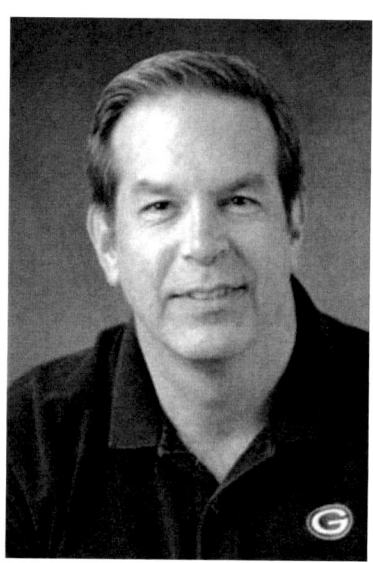

FOREWORD

"The best moments of our lives are not the passive, receptive, relaxing times...The best moments usually occur when a person's body or mind is stretched to its limits in a voluntary effort to accomplish something difficult and worthwhile. Optimal experience is thus something we make happen...In the long run it adds up to a sense of mastery—or perhaps better, a sense of participation in determining the content of life"—Mihaly Csikszentmihalyi

Grandmaster Hiang Kwang Thè has often told our martial arts class that there are three men who are the most influential people in his life: his father, Sek Heng Thè; his grandfather and primary martial arts teacher, Ie Chang Ming; and one of his other martial arts teachers, Liu Su Peng. For my greatest influence, it is easy. There's one: Hiang Kwang Thè.

I started training in martial arts in October of 1978 at the age of 25. I was wandering through the old Lexington Mall when I came across a table where Master Hiang Thè sat with brochures for his and his brother's new Sports Center, a huge, multi-discipline fitness facility that would be the precursor and model for many of today's modern health clubs. Though unassuming and low-key, you could sense he was a man of authenticity and quiet power.

I was seriously out-of-shape after a nearly six-month long post-college graduation road trip from one side of the country to the other spent sampling local potato chips and beer well before "buy local" became popular. Upon my return, I had begun a running program and was slowly melting off the pounds. In addition to a running track, weights, and a pool, Master Hiang's new place offered martial arts, something that had always piqued my interest after growing up in a neighborhood where you could get in a fight everyday if you walked or rode your bike down the wrong street or at the wrong time of the day. And I had been in a few. Unlike many of my smarter friends who would avoid those inevitable clashes by seeing who was at a playground before heading there or turning a deaf ear to insults shouted from neighborhood bullies, I just couldn't turn the other cheek. I was taught to never start a fight, but I wasn't going to run from anyone either, even if that meant getting my butt kicked from time to time.

So sign me up.

In each step of the way in my training with Master Hiang, I have learned so much from him through his martial arts teachings—physical fitness, mental toughness, self-defense, and especially the power of meditation and the internal arts. I loved his no-nonsense approach and his legendary demanding classes. More importantly, his teaching motivated me to be a better man. In addition to his great martial arts skill, I have seen first-hand how much he truly cares about his students, much more than he does financial gain or notoriety. Our long-term classes are much like families. Time after time, often with no one else's knowledge, he has been a true friend, supporter, and mentor when needed. He sets a great example of how to be there for friends and family.

Because of Master Hiang, I was also able to become an instructor, which has been one of the most rewarding facets of my life, to see my students grow and hopefully gain a few of the lessons Master Hiang passed on to me. Perhaps the greatest lesson taught was that having meaning in life, success, and self-awareness comes from one's own efforts. In 1978 I was too dependent on outside events, other people, and happenstance to bring me what I wanted out of life. But I learned from him that a meaningful, purposeful, well-lived life comes from one's own efforts. Not lotteries, not luck, not fate, not waiting for the phone to ring. Instead it comes from what we each put forth—towards the friendships we forge, the relationships we nurture, the people we inspire, the contributions we make. It wasn't the punch he taught me, but it was how to learn to punch. Not how to merely do a form, but what is behind it and what can you add to its meaning when you perform or teach it. Not just learning for my benefit, but to pass knowledge on to others. He'd love it if he saw you execute a perfect sweep on your classmate in sparring, but he'd be just as proud of you for putting out your hand to help your partner up.

And the greatest part of it all is that he has become one of my best and closest friends.

Little did I know in 1978 at that table in the mall how much my life would change for the better because of one man. The "nickname" given to him by his martial arts teachers is *Liu Fo Su* or "Sixth Sense Warrior." Maybe he already knew.

I am honored to be able to work with him on this book and video so that we can more widely share his vast knowledge on the subject and hopefully improve the lives of all those who will either be motivated to begin practicing Tai Chi or to gain greater insight into their own Tai Chi training. Please pass it on.

—*Master David Cubine, 2017*

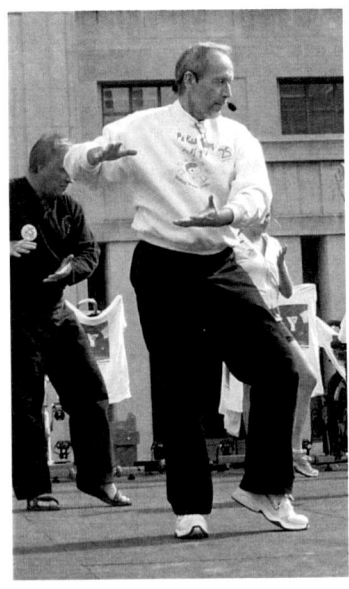

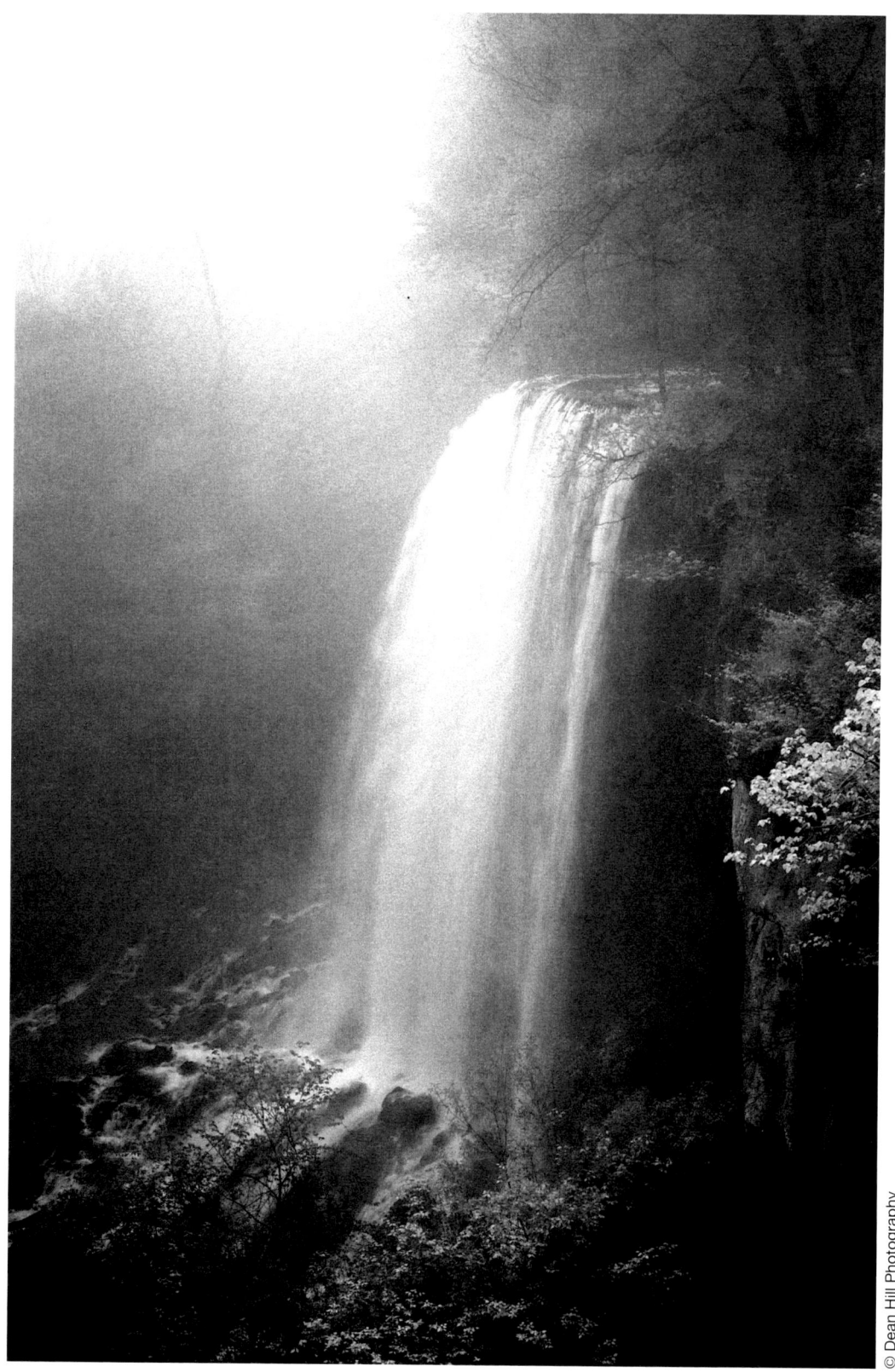

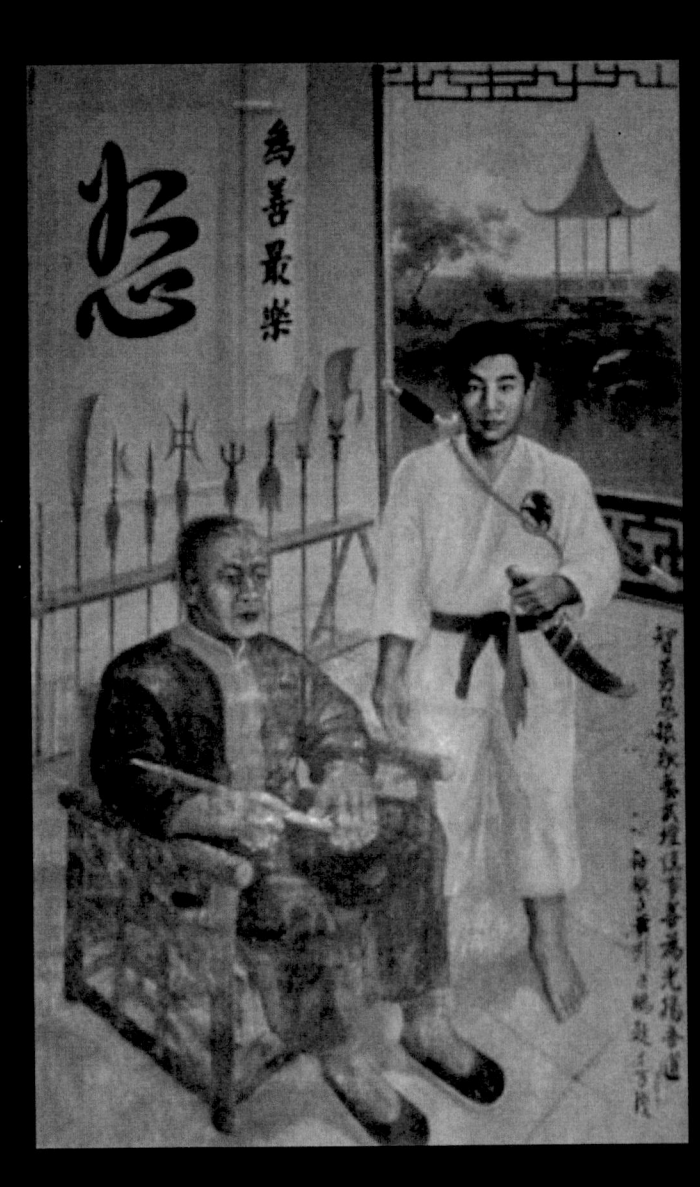

PREFACE

WHILE GROWING UP IN BANDUNG, INDONESIA, I frequently visited the shop of my grandfather, Ie Chang Ming, which was just a few blocks away. He had a studio there where he practiced and taught martial arts. Even before he allowed me to start taking his classes at age eight, I would still watch and act out the movements I saw him and the others practicing.

He was also known by the name T'ieh Chang Shang Ren or the "Iron Palm Master." His abilities with the internal or Nei Kung side of martial arts were exceptional. We occasionally heard stories about his days in China from others—about the places where and people with whom he studied—but he was a humble and reserved man who did not boast of his abilities or exploits. He didn't have to. It was obvious to anyone who watched him that he was very highly skilled.

My grandfather was very particular to whom he taught martial arts. It was by invitation only and he liked to know the families of the students he did select. During much of the later years of my training, there was quite a bit of political unrest in the country and, being Chinese, my family kept a low profile. It was the same with our practice of martial arts.

I often practiced six days a week, both before and after school. I loved it so much, plus I got to be with my grandfather. I started training with the internal forms around age 10, then progressed to learning Lee Family Tai Chi three or four years later once I had matured enough. When he saw that I put in extra effort and time to practice it, he offered special instruction to me for Tai Chi and the other internal studies. I know he pushed me harder than most of the others. Maybe it was because I was his grandson, or because I was the youngest or smallest person in the class. But he knew that the additional attention would not be wasted on me. I loved it and was dedicated to my practice.

My grandfather's teaching style was based on one important principal—learn to learn for yourself. He followed the adage described in the old proverb "Give a man a fish and you feed him for a day. Teach a man to fish and you feed him for a lifetime." He did not like to show things again and again or repeat something he had already told us. He expected us to pay attention during class, do our homework, and figure out ways to remember what he had taught us. He also encouraged my classmates and me to work together on our own to "brainstorm" on the material he showed us. One of my grandfather's favorite things to say to us was, "Think," that the answer is already there in front of us. As long as we were putting in the effort, he would guide us in the right direction if we weren't on the right track. Although he ran his classes with discipline, he was a kind and patient man, and our improvement was his main goal.

My grandfather encouraged us to be strong, but also to be kind. For us to keep a clear mind, be calm, and when faced with adversity, be brave. I carried those lessons with me when I left home to travel halfway around the world in August of 1968 to the United States, the place that would become my new home and where I would become a proud citizen and raise a family of my own. Since then I have tried to impart those lessons to my students and to my own children and grandchildren. I hope I have had some small amount of success.

This book and video are the result of my strong desire to improve people's lives by sharing my knowledge of the lifelong study of Lee Family Tai Chi as taught to me by my grandfather. Before I left home, he told me, "Don't forget this one," referring to Lee Family Tai Chi. As anyone who knows me can tell you, I like to avoid over-promising or hyping anything. The truth is that practicing Lee Family Tai Chi has certainly improved my life in a profound way. I am convinced that it will also improve yours.

My grandfather, Ie Chang Ming, passed away in 1968. I am dedicating this book to his memory.

Hiang Kwang Thè—2017

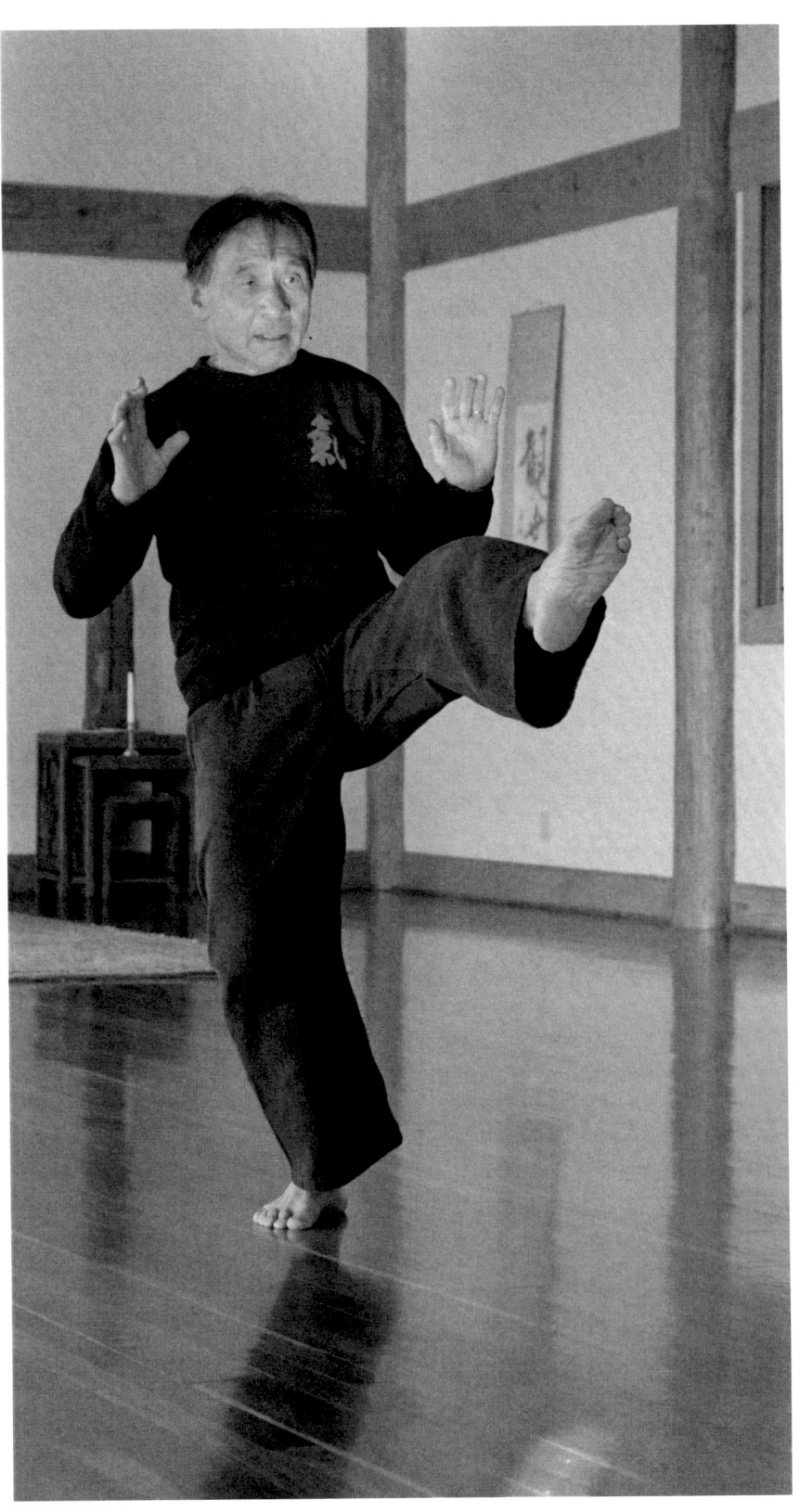

ONE

INTRODUCTION: WHAT IS LEE FAMILY TAI CHI?

NOW, MORE THAN EVER, WE ALL NEED TO FIND A WAY TO BRING BALANCE INTO OUR LIVES. From career, family, and social demands to the increased volume and way we receive information, the pace of modern life can easily overcome our abilities to cope in a healthy way. So where do we look for this balance in current times? I believe one of the best sources can be found in the past.

For most of my life, I have practiced Lee Family Tai Chi. Tai Chi was an integral part of my martial arts training that began at the age of eight with my grandfather, Grandmaster Ie Chang Ming. As most young people do, I was more interested in the active, physical side of the training or "bouncing off the walls" as I like to tell my students now. But as I grew older, I started to realize the importance of what we call the "internal" side of the practice, including Tai Chi.

If you asked me to write a definition of Tai Chi for the dictionary, it might read something like this: Tai Chi is an exercise system that consists of several linked movements, performed slowly and continuously, in tandem with controlled breathing techniques, based on a philosophy of achieving harmony, unification, and balance. Tai Chi trains us to think and move as "one" while developing a greater awareness of mind, body, and spirit—a great *inner balance*.

The Great Balancing

In short, I like to describe Tai Chi practice as the "Great Balancing." The full name of the style we practice is Lee Chia Tai Chi Chuan or the Lee Family Tai Chi Form. Some descriptions of Tai Chi Chuan use terms like "meditation in motion" or more literal translations like the martial arts sounding "Grand Ultimate Fist." Those are accurate labels, but I like the "Great Balancing" as I believe that the Lee Family form is more focused on health rather than martial arts. In fact, the translation of the "Chi" character in Tai Chi can be as a pole or an axis, as in the North Pole (Pei Chi) or South Pole (Nan Chi), the axis upon which the earth rotates in balance. In my opinion, Lee Family Tai Chi helps you more effectively create a balance of inner calm, energy/Chi flow, equilibrium, and awareness than any other exercise program. The focus of this book and video is using Lee Family Tai Chi for the Ultimate Health.

Don't Forget This One

One of the most important pieces of advice I received from my grandfather was him telling me "not to forget this one" just before I left my home in Bandung, Indonesia for the United States in 1968. He was referring to Lee Family Tai Chi. Grandmaster Ie and my other teachers at his school all practiced Lee Family Tai Chi daily and often as a warm-up for or cool-down from their other martial arts training. His words and actions have left a strong imprint on both my own practice and on my approach to teaching since then.

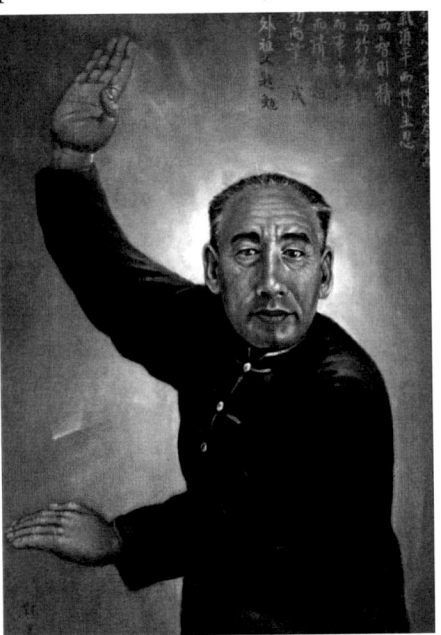
My grandfather and teacher, Ie Chang Ming

I initially only taught Lee Family Tai Chi to my advanced martial arts students. Part of that was because Tai Chi and other meditative arts were not very well known or practiced in western culture

Lee Family Tai Chi Chuan

when I started teaching in the United States in 1968. The way they had often been presented up to that point was as something mystical—unproven by western science—and I didn't want to come across as a "snake oil salesman" to those who had not been exposed to this type of study. My advanced students had already experienced the benefits of internal, or "Nei Kung" training and we also applied the principles of Tai Chi's use of force and heightened awareness in our sparring, so I kept it in-house for many years.

Gradually, the benefits of meditation became more widespread. Studies from well-respected science and medical institutions began to emerge and, just as importantly, people sought better ways to deal with stress, aching joints, mental issues, and aging. I cautiously began to offer Tai Chi and other internal classes like Chi Kung to non-martial arts students. I quickly realized that not only was there a great demand for this type of knowledge, but I was able to directly see the health benefits in action outside of the martial arts classroom.

So what are some of these benefits? Improvements in:

- Core postural strength
- Physical balance
- Flexibility
- Memory loss and dementia
- Rheumatoid arthritis
- Type 2 diabetes
- COPD
- Hypertension

Studies have also shown that Tai Chi practice can:

- increase our ability to handle stress
- help reduce unwanted side effects of chemotherapy and radiation
- help prevent falls in older adults
- slow the effects of osteoarthritis
- improve abilities of those with Parkinson's disease
- help fight depression and anxiety

In much older times in China, before modern medicine, Chi Kung practices were one of the few ways that people could treat illnesses and injury. As it was then, Tai Chi can also be a type of diagnostic tool that lets you know where problems are developing, so you can put more emphasis there in your training or choose to see a physician.

Of course, there are no magical cures and we are all born with our own genetic predisposition, which may make us more susceptible to certain health problems. We do have the choice, however, to improve the genetic "hand we are dealt" by maintaining a healthy lifestyle, diet, exercising and working on our emotional and mental well-being. I believe that Lee Family Tai Chi is a great way to achieve those goals. As I tell my classes, if you can do Lee Tai Chi in the morning, you are not going to "go down" that day.

Other Benefits

There are several Tai Chi family styles practiced today. These are some of the practical benefits to the Lee Family Tai Chi's particular style.

- It does not require a lot of floor space to perform. We often use a circular shape to describe the practice area. The diameter of this circular boundary is about the same as the person's height. For example, a six-foot man would cover a circular area about six feet in diameter. You don't have to move furniture and can even do it in a hotel room if you are traveling.

- It doesn't require a long time commitment, so it is easier to incorporate into our busy lifestyles. The Lee Family form can be done in 12-15 minutes depending upon the pace. And if you desire a longer practice time, the Lee Family form's duration is easily doubled by just repeating the form.

- Through practice, you can develop the ability to focus or "target" your vital organs or other areas of your body to improve either specific health issues or your overall wellness.

You Will Be Rewarded

During my time teaching Lee Family Tai Chi, the number one request from my students has been to produce a book and a video to aid in the practice and understanding of this excellent exercise system. After many years of effort towards its creation, I am now proud to be able to offer them to you.

People of all ages, both men and women, and individuals with a range of physical abilities and health issues, attend my classes. I don't believe Tai Chi discriminates. I would love to be able to go back in time and ask its creators what it was that they were thinking when they developed Lee Family Tai Chi. Even though I don't know exactly what they would say, I am convinced that they wanted to find a way to improve the lives of others in what was surely a rugged time to live. I also think they asked a lot of those to whom they taught it—to spend the time, the effort and the energy it would take to acquire something of value. I strongly believe that if you invest *your* time in practicing Lee Family Tai Chi, you too will be rewarded.

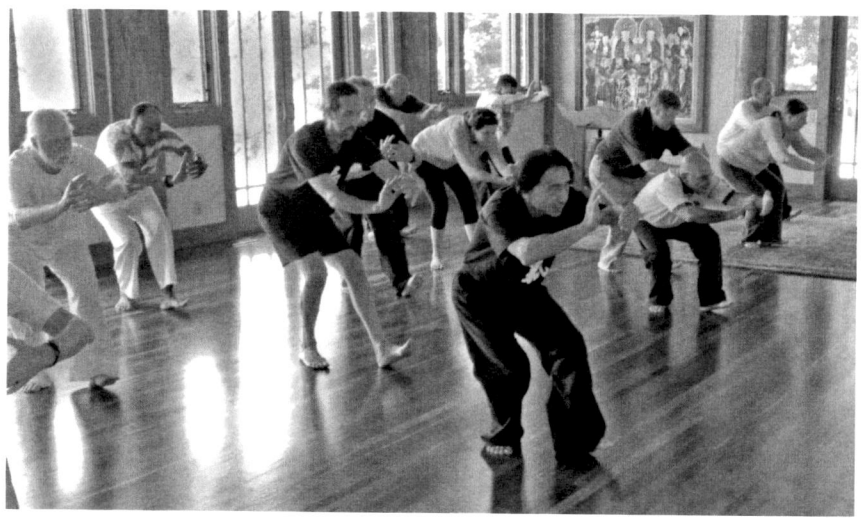

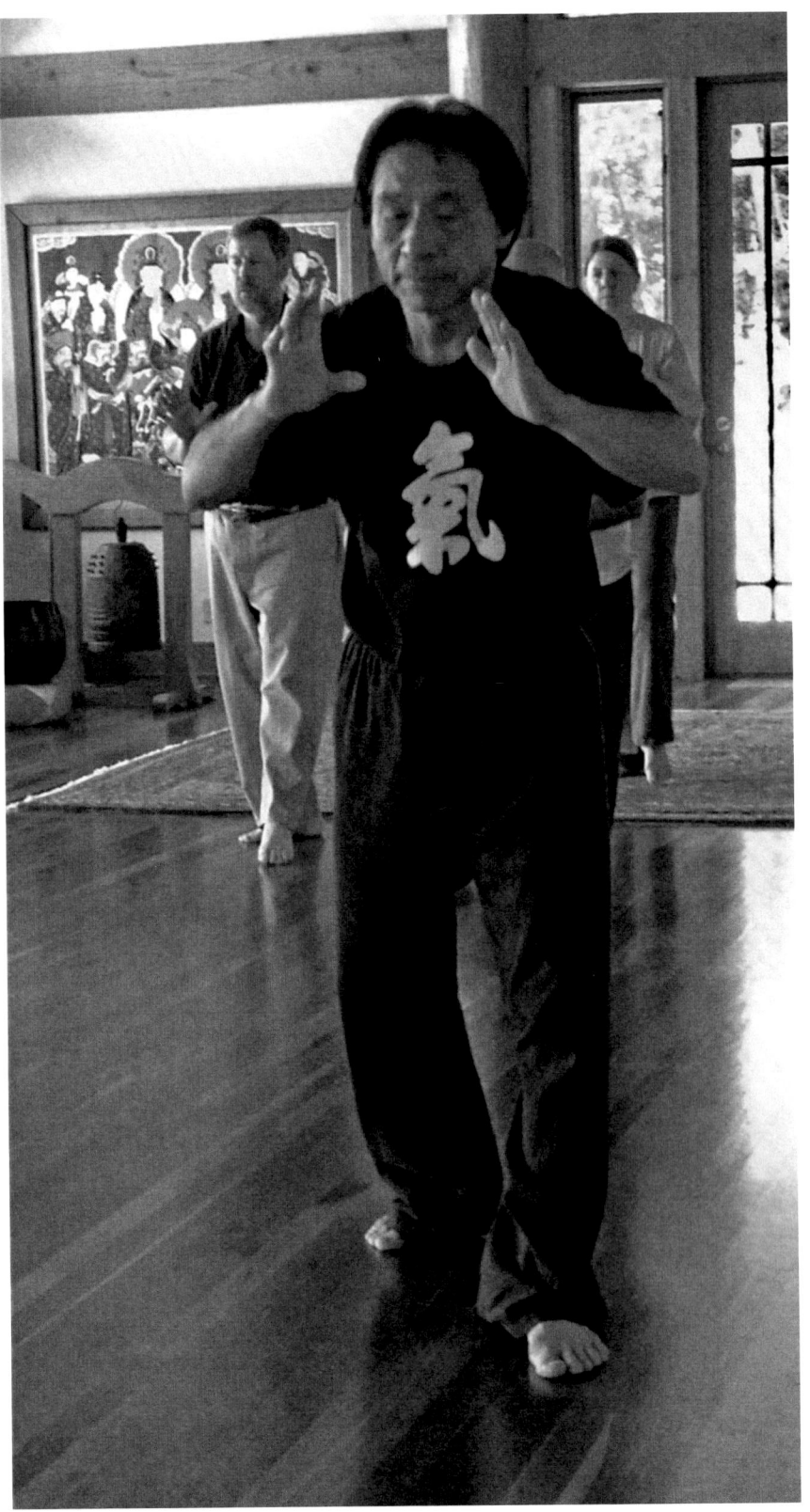

TWO

HOW TO USE THIS BOOK AND VIDEO

THIS BOOK AND THE COMPANION VIDEO ARE INTENDED TO SERVE TWO MAIN PURPOSES: The first is to offer Lee Family Tai Chi to a much broader audience—those who are not able to take a class with us to learn in person. The second is to give all practitioners a much greater depth of understanding about Lee Family Tai Chi and how to achieve the most benefit from its practice.

Learning The Form

I recommend putting your initial efforts into learning the form itself. The form section of this book contains photographs of each of the 60 postures, both the inhale/Yin side and exhale/Yang portion, and gives a brief description of the movements. While the still images are helpful for reviewing, making corrections and adjustments in your form, or to better help learn the sequence of moves, they do not give as good of an idea of the transitions between the movements or the flow. Viewing or practicing along with the video is the primary way to begin to learn the form.

Video

We have divided the Form portion of the video into a Complete Form section and an Individual Posture section. In the Complete Form section, I do the entire form, from beginning to end, without stopping. The complete form section includes an overhead view to help you determine where you are within the circular shape of the form's boundary. We also include the letters "I" and "E"— I for inhale and E for exhale— in the upper left corner to indicate the breathing sequence.

Viewing the complete form is very helpful in getting an understanding of the flow, pace, and breathing sequence. You can do the form along with me almost as if I were in the room with you giving you cues as you learn the complete sequence. We have a version with no narration and a version with me calling out the complete form as I would if we were doing it together in a class. Use this audio portion if having my voice as a cue helps you go through the form rather than just watching a video screen alone.

In the Individual Posture Section, we have divided the form into 11 smaller sections. Each of the individual sections is similar in length to a single one-hour class in a 12-week session when Lee Family Tai Chi is taught in person. (The last class of each session is used for review.) In each of these, I go through the movements several times and detail the points of emphasis of those movements. Beginning students should practice one section at a time, in sequence, until you feel comfortable with that section's movements, before moving on to the next section. Students learning in-person can use each section for review between each week's class. For those who have been through the complete form, each section can also be used to study the movements in greater detail and work on the stances, equilibrium, and breathing. When just learning the form, it is natural for your focus to be mainly on remembering the physical movements—turn left, turn right, extend the left hand, etc.—so going back and reviewing each section can help you discover other aspects of the form that may have been missed the first time through.

The beginning of the Individual Posture Section also includes more detail about some of the fundamentals of your practice. In the first part, we review Stances, Transfer of Weight, and Equilibrium. In the second, Breathing and Pace, we discuss the proper breathing techniques and the pace of movement you should maintain throughout the form. These topics are also covered in the book.

We wrap up the video with an interview where I answer some of the most frequently asked questions from students.

Book

Roots, Philosophy and Foundation: The book does contain information not included in the video. In the first third of the book, I review some of Tai Chi's history, background and roots. We explore some of the benefits of practicing Tai Chi and how to reap the greatest health rewards. We also examine what is behind the practice, its philosophy, the meaning of Yin and Yang, and the concept of Chi.

The Form: The middle section of the book is focused on the form itself. As mentioned above, we include photos of the entire form, in sequence, showing both the Inhale/Yin and Exhale/Yang portion of the 60 postures along with a brief text description of the movements. We also include what vital organ is in play with each posture, which is detailed in the Targeting chapter of the book.

Hows and Whys: In the last third of the book, we consider how to get the most out of the practice. We go into detail about the Stances, Weight Transfer, Equilibrium, proper Breathing, and Targeting. We also offer some guidance with practice tips and present a number of training exercises and routines that can be done outside of the form itself to greatly improve your skill level and awareness.

FAQs: We have also included the answers to a number of the most frequently asked questions I receive during classes. Student questions over the years have proven to be an extremely valuable asset in developing our teaching strategy and have influenced what material we cover in this book and video. This is also a quick way to review a list of some of the more important points made throughout the book's text.

Beginner, Intermediate and Advanced

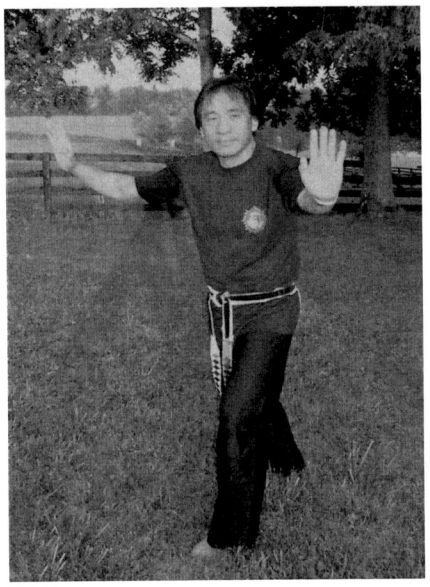

We have written the text so that the beginning, intermediate, and advanced student can all gain knowledge. For the beginning student, some of the more in-depth material may not be as understandable upon initial reading of the book. We have attempted to introduce basic concepts wherever possible for the beginner at the start of the chapters, then go into more depth as the chapters continue for the more experienced student. So a beginner may find that they will want to either re-read or save the later parts of certain sections for when they have more experience. The intermediate student will find the more in-depth information as a way to open the door to deeper understanding, hopefully switching on that mental light bulb and inspiring them to dig even deeper. The more advanced student may find the information presented as the path to even greater understanding and refinement of the skills already acquired.

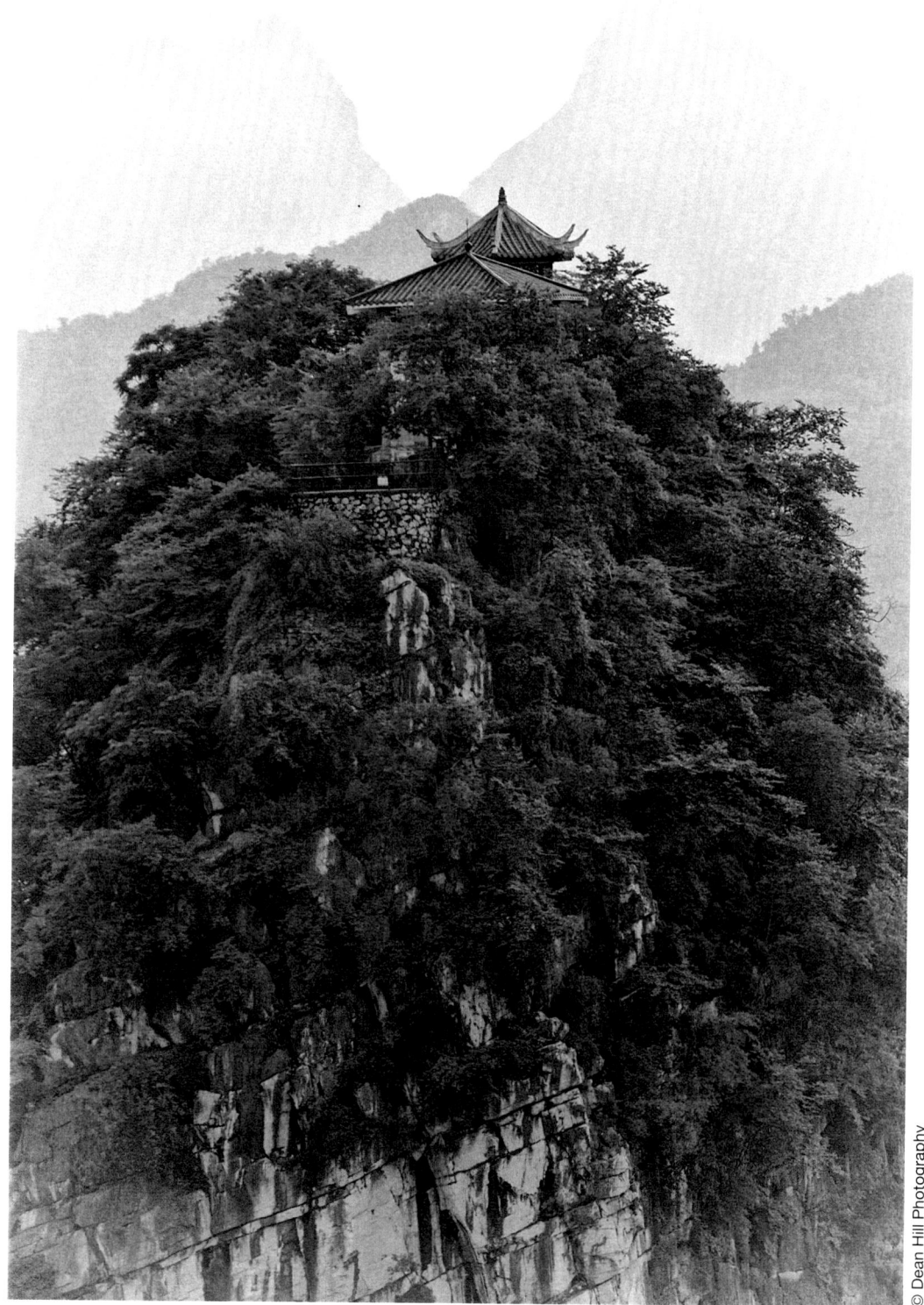

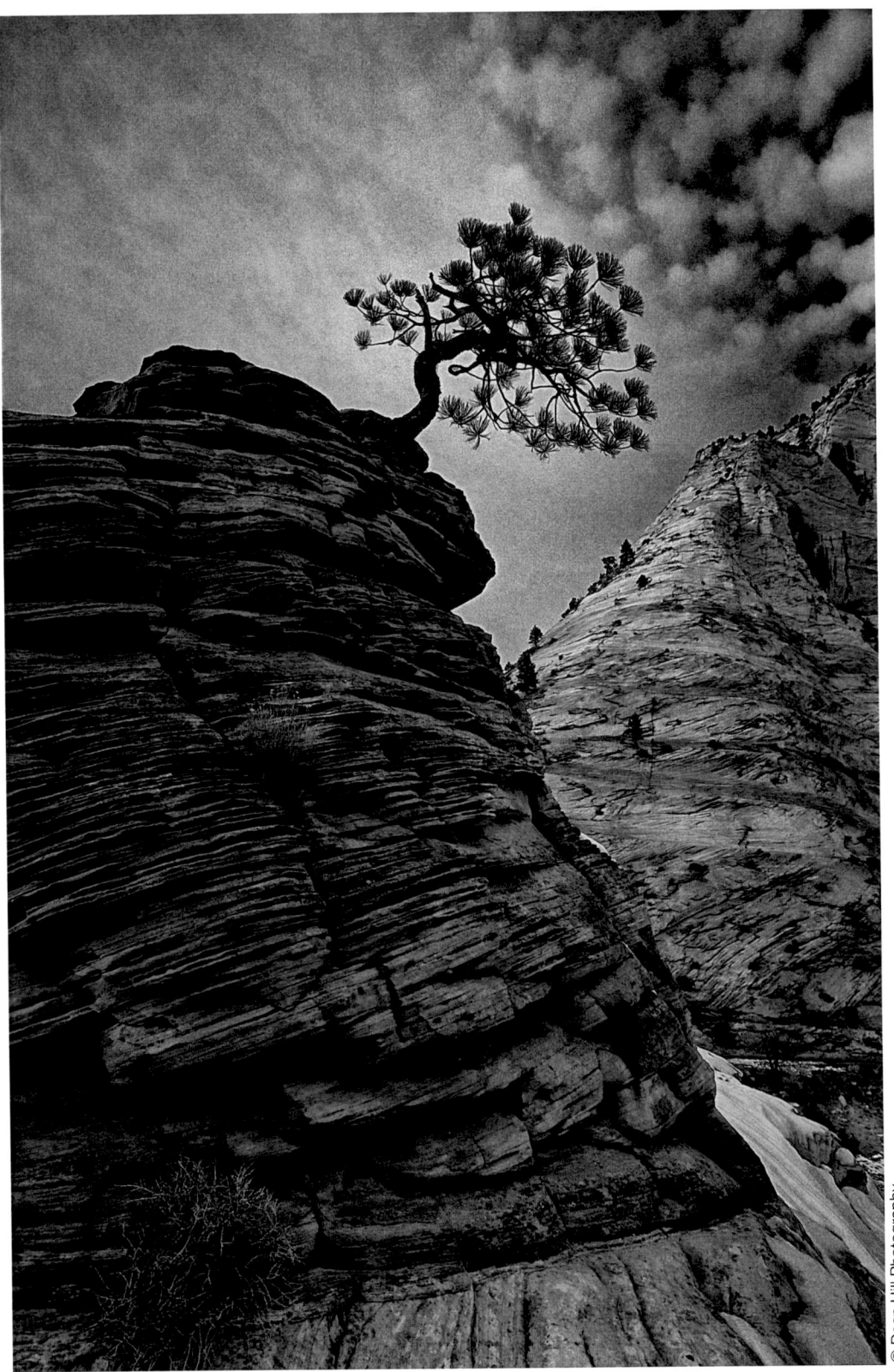

THREE

ROOTS

I DO NOT KNOW EXACTLY WHEN LEE FAMILY TAI CHI WAS CREATED, but I can say with confidence that it is very old, perhaps 1000 years or more, with its roots going even farther back in time. My grandfather, who taught me Lee Famliy Tai Chi, did not discuss the history of it with me. I wish I had asked more about it, but at the time, being young and out of respect, I usually waited for him to let me know about such things.

Research from 2005 did uncover some previously undocumented Lee (Li) Family genealogy at the Qianzai Temple in Henan, China. The research showed that around the year 1650, members of the Lee Family developed what they called "The Art of Tai Chi Cultivating Life" and "The Thirteen Postures Boxing." Other research shows that a Qianzai Temple priest named Shi Lee (Li) developed a Tai Chi-like system based on earlier Chi Kung exercises sometime in the 7th century. A stone inscription from him reads, *"Don't be bully of futileness, the pugilism is for life and health. The softness overcomes the hardness, give up yourself and follow the opponent."*

Much of Chinese history is oral and the recorded ancestry may have been destroyed or lost. I can hypothesize that by comparing Lee Family Tai Chi, its postures, and its internal work with the other Chi Kung practices at that time and with later Tai Chi family styles, that the Lee Family form was probably developed sometime during or around the early Sung Dynasty which began in 960 AD.

A Brief History

At the time of the Sung Dynasty in Chinese history, many Chi Kung or internal energy practices were quickly emerging. Even well before that though, the roots of what would become Lee Family Tai Chi were also being developed.

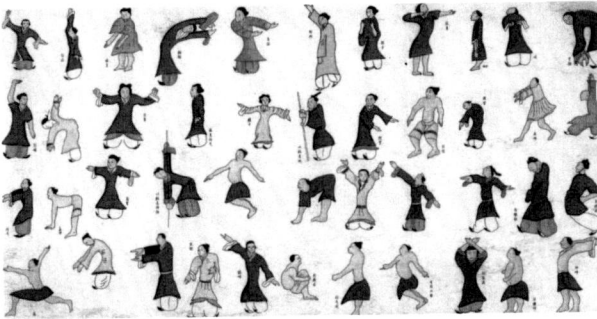

Tao Yin Tu painting from the Mawangui Scroll depicts Chi Kung exercises from around 200BC

The first records of Chinese medicine emerged during the rule of the Yellow Emperor, Huang Ti (2690-2590 BC). The landmark *I Ching/Book of Changes* was written soon after. It introduced the concept of Chi and established a philosophy based on the natural order of forces in nature, which runs deep in Chinese culture. A scroll from the Mawangdui Tomb in China circa 200 BC called "Tao Yin Tu" depicts movements and breathing exercises for circulating Chi.

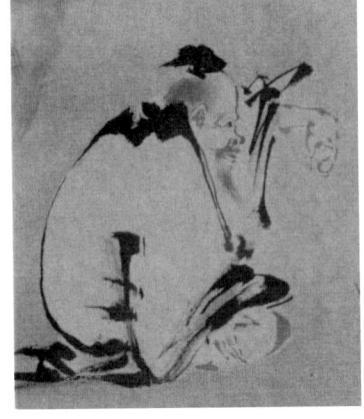

During the 6th century BC, Lao Tzu (Lee Earl) was believed to have birthed Taoism and the concept of Yin and Yang as the guiding laws of the universe in his *Tao Te Ching* or "The Way" —in effect, the "Great Balance of Nature." The text studies the human spirit, nature, and inner reflection. It is also believed to be the first recorded use of breathing to strengthen Chi. The Taoists also practiced combining breathing, massage, and meditation to create an "alchemy" or transformation of these separate parts to create and circulate Chi.

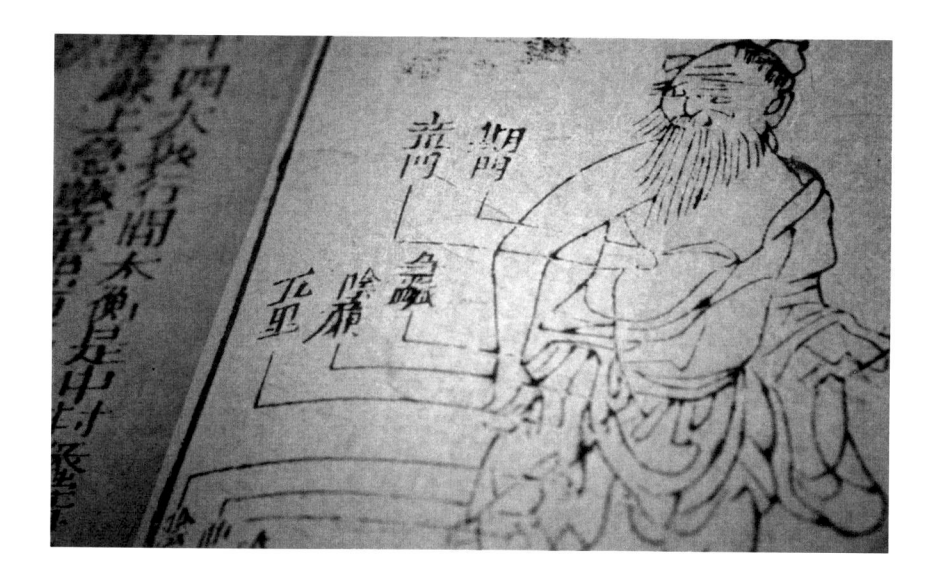

The practice of acupuncture also started around this time, expanding on the ideas of Chi flow by discovering meridians and vessels, the body's Chi paths and storage areas, and how to manipulate those paths externally with needles.

Then in the 6th century AD, a Buddhist monk named Bodhidharma arrived at the Shaolin Temple in China's Henan province. Bodhidharma is credited with developing a Chi Kung exercise program to help strengthen and improve the health of the monks called *Yi Chin Ching* or "Muscle Development Classic." This program was later incorporated into the temple's martial arts training. It is believed that these were the beginnings of the use of Chi Kung in the practice of martial arts.

There is some evidence of other Tai Chi-like systems being practiced in the time of the Tang Dynasty (618-905 AD) and Liang Dynasty (907-921 AD). These records show internal training being done with individual postures that would later be linked together referencing some of the principals of the I Ching's "eight trigrams" and "five elements" that are fundamental to Tai Chi. Some of the movements even had names that would be used in later Tai Chi forms like "grasp the sparrow's tail." More evidence may emerge from this period with further study.

Buddhism, Confucianism, and Taoism

To give a frame of reference to this varied history, there were three main schools of philosophy at the time: Buddhism, Confucianism, and Taoism. As it relates to Chi Kung practice, Buddhism was largely concerned with reducing suffering through greater awareness. The Confucians were more concerned with one's intellect and improving a person's function in society. The Taoists emphasized enlightenment, health, and immortality working with the balance of nature. The Taoists also believed in the idea of "soft" over "hard" and worked with the body's center or Tan Tien as our source of Chi, which are essential parts of current Tai Chi practice. What we then have later with Tai Chi practice—with its foundation based on a balance of body, mind, and spirit—may have developed out of a synthesis of the Taoist, Buddhism and Confucian traditions.

The principals of Lee Family Tai Chi all follow and have their roots in these early studies, and as a result, it may have been developed close to this early time in the Sung Dynasty when the internal arts were exploding.

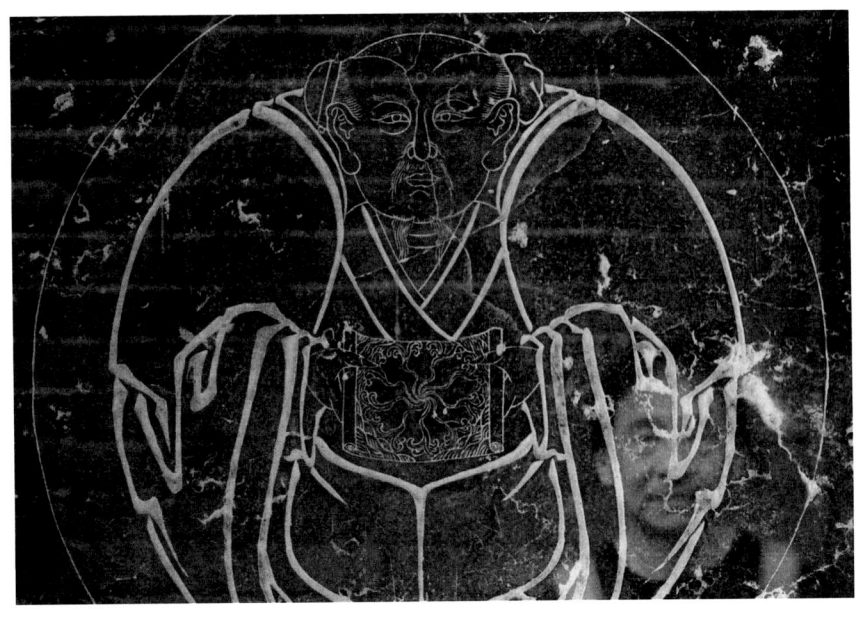

Stone tablet from the Henan Shaolin Temple representing the combination of Taoist, Buddhist and Confucian teachings.

DID YOU KNOW?

Tai Chi or Tai Chi Chuan?

For the purpose of this book, we have used the term *Tai Chi* to describe the exercise regimen and form we are practicing. To clarify, the full name of the exercise system is often written as Tai Chi Chuan, translated as the "Supreme Ultimate Fist/Boxing," which belies its martial arts application in many cases. The "Tai Chi" referenced in the Philosophy chapter is the path from Wu Chi, and describes the idea of the ultimate source of the universe and creation, from which spring Yin and Yang, and upon which Tai Chi Chuan practice is based. In that chain of creation events, there are additional levels of evolution described: Yin and Yang are followed by the Five Elements, then Pa Kua's Eight Trigrams, and then the 64 Hexagrams.

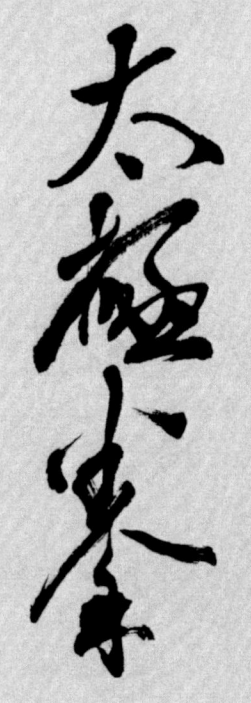

Tai- "Great" or "supreme." Combines three individual characters. Top straight line means "one," middle character is "person," and bottom dot is "centered," or "One Centered Person Between Heaven and Earth."

Chi- This Chi refers to balance. Combines the character on the left of a pine tree, as "relaxed as a pine tree" with the compound character on the right of the mouth and hand split by a center line representing "Uses the Hand and the Mouth in a Balanced Fashion on Earth."

Chuan- Often translated as "fist" or "boxing," relating to Tai Chi's martial arts applications, but is also used in the word "earnest" or "sincere" or "to roll up one's sleeves and bare one's fists being eager to get started."

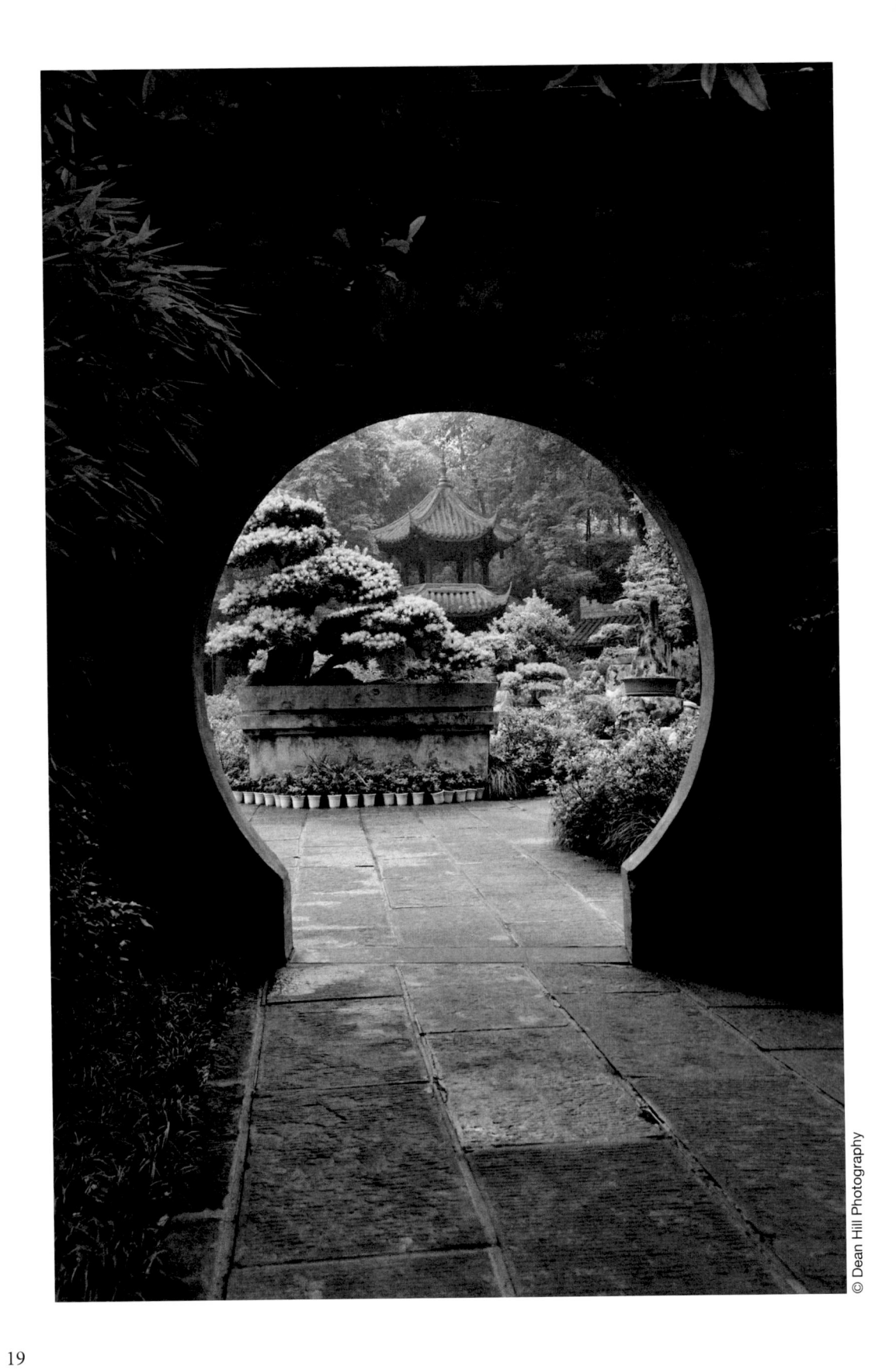

FOUR

PHILOSOPHY & FOUNDATION

Chi

THE CONCEPT OF CHI IS A BIT ELUSIVE because it doesn't have a real definition in the west. To the eastern culture, Chi (pronounced "chee") is defined as one's vital or life force—the energy in all living things. Like electricity or water, it can flow, circulate, be diverted, increase or decrease in strength, and can be released or blocked. Like electricity, we may not be able to see it, but we can certainly feel it and notice its results on our health. The concept most closely related to Chi in the west is the idea of "bio-electricity." The early Chinese writings on the subject also relate Chi to the blood, saying, "where the Chi goes, the blood will follow."

Chi Kung

Chi Kung (Qigong) is the training system we use to develop our Chi. Tai Chi is a type of Chi Kung practice. Chi Kung is translated as "Energy Work," so through this practice, we can work with and develop our Chi, or vital life force, to use for a number of purposes. We all are born with Chi. The other sources of Chi are in the food and liquids we consume, from the air we breathe, from the earth, and from the celestial bodies. So a healthy diet, clean air, and spending time outdoors are all great ways to gather as much Chi as we can. More importantly, we can also work within ourselves to improve our Chi. One of the main goals of Tai Chi training is to cultivate the Chi in three ways:

- Increase the *amount* of Chi
- Increase the *quality* of Chi
- Increase the *circulation* of Chi

The number one way to achieve these three goals is through your effort. The more you practice, the greater the Chi development. You will also become more sensitive to this growth and be much better able to feel your Chi at work.

Meridians and Vessels

Our human body is made up of a number of systems—circulatory, pulmonary, nervous, lymphatic, digestive, skeletal, endocrine, muscular, renal, reproductive—all connected and communicating with one another. Traditional Chinese Medicine also recognizes a system of Chi flow that lays the body out like a series of rivers, streams and reservoirs. These are called meridians and vessels.

We have 12 meridians that circulate our Chi through the body and extend out to the limbs and extremities on one end, and connect to the body's major organs on the other end. Six are considered Yin and six are considered Yang (see Yin-Yang, page 26). These 12 meridians are also duplicated on each side of the body in a mirror image.

We also have eight vessels that carry and store our Chi, like a reservoir. Think of these vessels as a battery or capacitor used for energy storage. The vessels also help to regulate the flow of Chi in the meridians. Two of the eight vessels are: 1) The Conception Vessel, that runs along a center line of the front of the torso from the upper lip to the perineum;

DID YOU KNOW?

Chi and Chi Kung Chinese Characters

The traditional Chinese logograph for *Chi Kung* or "Energy Work" tells an interesting story. It combines the elements of life—air, food, fire, and water—and, more importantly, the energy created from their combination. Practicing Chi Kung is developing the skills necessary to create or "cultivate" energy through one's strong efforts.

CHI

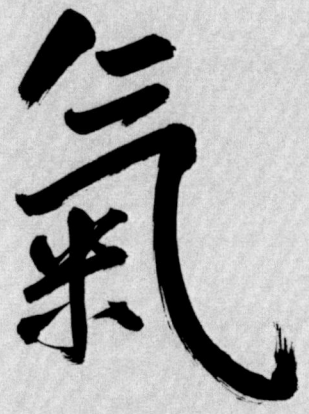

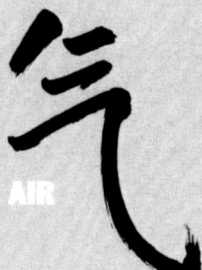

氣　气　米

AIR — The top section refers to the air we breathe. Placed on top to indicate its importance.

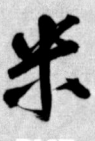

RICE — Rice grain is grown with water and prepared with fire. Energy is created from the combustion.

KUNG

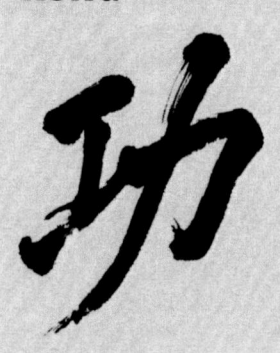

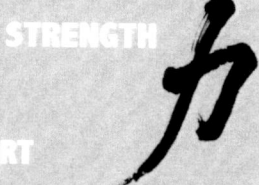

功　工　力

EFFORT — The "I" shape on the left is work or effort.

STRENGTH — The shape on the right is Li, to have strength.

Combined, they mean skill or ability. It takes effort to acquire skill.

Philosophy & Foundation

and 2) The Governing Vessel, that runs along a center line of the back of the torso from the perineum, around the top of the head, and to the upper lip. The two vessels are attached at the two end points to form a circular path called the Small Circulation or Small Heavenly Circle. Together, the Conception Vessel and Governing Vessel form the most important Chi reservoir in the body.

The other six vessels are the Thrusting Vessel, the Girdle Vessel, the Yang Heel Vessel, the Yin Heel Vessel, the Yang Linking Vessel, and the Yin Linking Vessel. When you focus and guide your Chi out to the arms and legs through these vessels in a particular larger pathway, the route is called the Grand Circulation. (See the Targeting chapter for more details on circulating Chi outside of the Small Circulation.) We hope to explore these aspects in greater depth in future volumes.

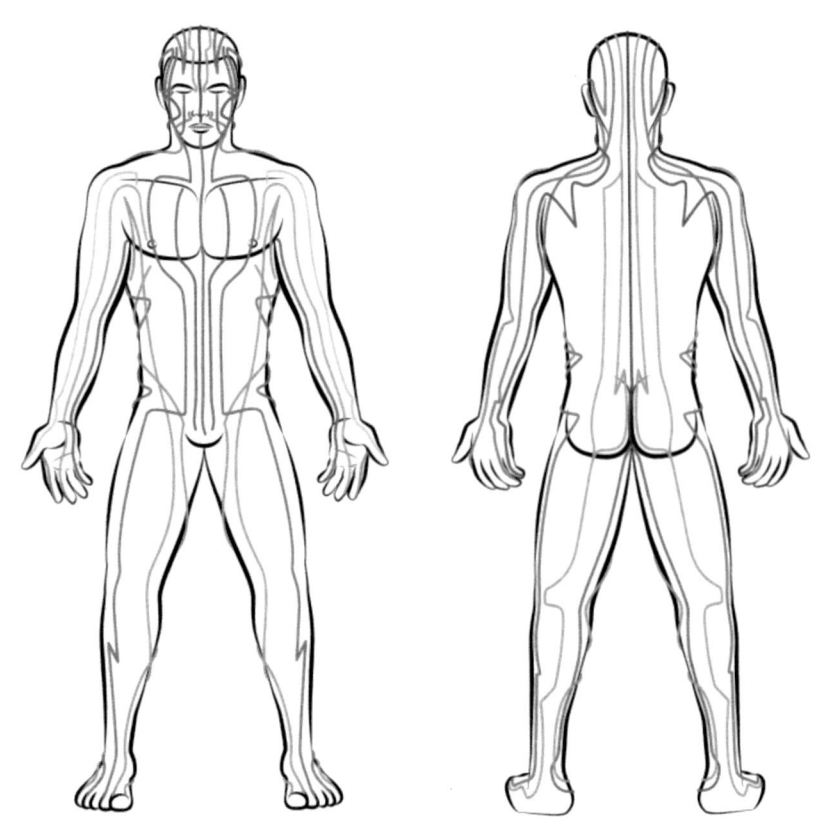

Meridians and Vessels

The Tan Tien or "main point/field" referenced elsewhere in this book is also found along the path of the Conception Vessel around one to two inches below the navel. Other important points or "cavities" are at various places along this circular path, but the Tan Tien is considered the original source of a person's energy and is a key focal point for Tai Chi practice.

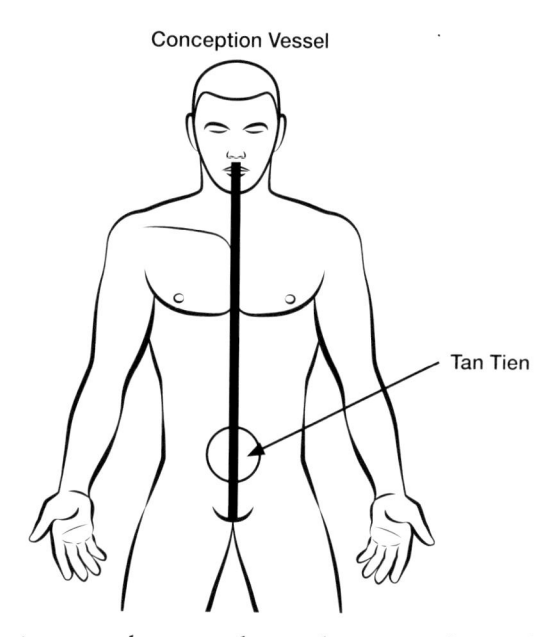

By concentrating on these paths and points along the paths while doing our focused breathing—and our movements in the case of Tai Chi—we are able to fill them with Chi so that they open up and circulate the Chi smoothly throughout the body without stagnation, bathing all the major organs and reaching out to the extremities. We want these channels to remain open and flowing, without choking off our Chi flow.

You can relate this Chi system layout and function to a gas furnace in your home. You bring in air, combine it with fuel, and light it with a spark to create heat that the fan and ductwork take to the rooms in your house. The more efficient the system, the better your home is heated and the lower your fuel costs. So you breathe in an efficient and controlled way, light the fire in your Tan Tien area, and then circulate your Chi with your mind through the vessels and meridians.

The Yie

Your mind? Yes, the *mind leads the Chi.* The other important component in this system is how you guide your Chi along these paths and to the areas where you want to place your Chi—think of your mind as the computer that commands the system and operates the controls. Chinese culture has two names for the mind—the Yie (pronounced "ee") and Hsin (pronounced "sin"). The Hsin is your heart or more feeling side. Affected by the emotions, it is also more passive. Hsin is sometimes referred to as the "naughty" or "mischievous mind" in that it is considered the part of the mind that may try to talk you out of doing the right thing or putting forth proper effort. It can be the unwanted noise or chatter that is getting in the way of having a clear mind.

The Yie is your intent or will. It is also related to wisdom and judgment, and is more active. In Chi Kung, *you use your entire conscious mind, your Yie, to help guide your Chi.* When your mind has a thought, your Yie strives to make it happen. The Yie is focused and firmed by the will. If you want to direct your Chi out to your hands, then you use your Yie to guide it there. If you want to get more Chi to your heart, then it's your Yie that is running the show. (See the Targeting chapter for more details on guiding Chi to your vital organs.) And because the use of the mind is important in Chi Kung, we want to also develop a harmony of Hsin and Yie in our general make-up for the most balanced state of mind.

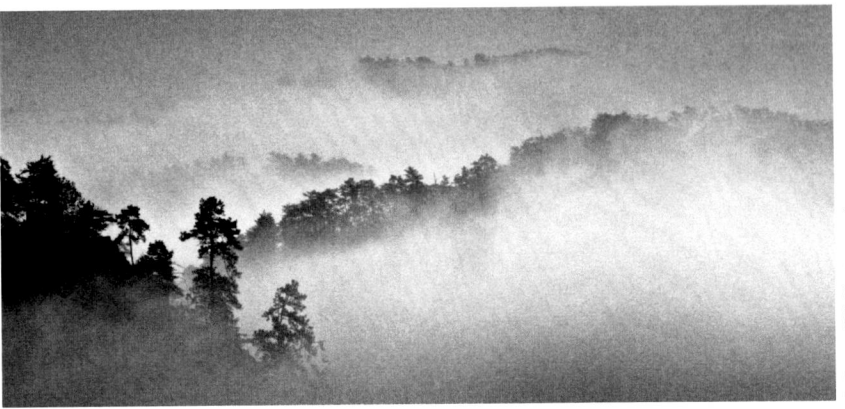

Yin and Yang

Taoist philosophers in ancient China believed that the natural universe was bound by the laws of opposites—Yin and Yang. These beliefs spawned an entire school of thought with principals and ideas that still run deep in the fiber of Chinese culture. This subject is complex, with a number of layers to dissect in order to fully comprehend. But I think a brief discussion is important, as this concept is fundamental to the development and practice of Tai Chi.

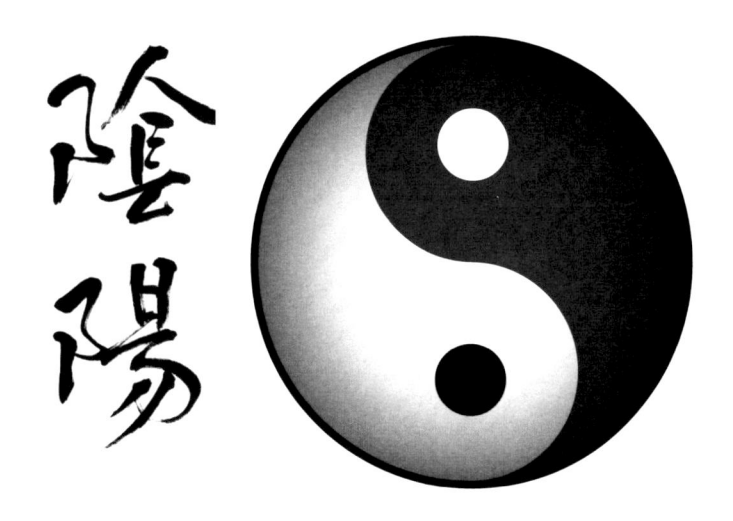

So where did this Yin and Yang idea originate? These early philosophers created a linear flow chart of sorts to describe what they believed were the origins of the universe and explain the natural structure and balance of events. It began with what was called "Wu Chi," or a formless state of pure nothingness. Wu Chi evolved into "Tai Chi," or the "Grand Terminus"—the starting point for existence (see illustration, next page). Philosopher Lao Tzu (also named Lee Earl, as it is believed by many researchers) the author credited with writing the seminal *I Ching,* or "Book of Changes," called this concept "The Tao," which translates as "The Way" or "The Path." Tai Chi then evolved into Yin and Yang, "…and then came everything else," said Lao Tzu.

Philosophy & Foundation

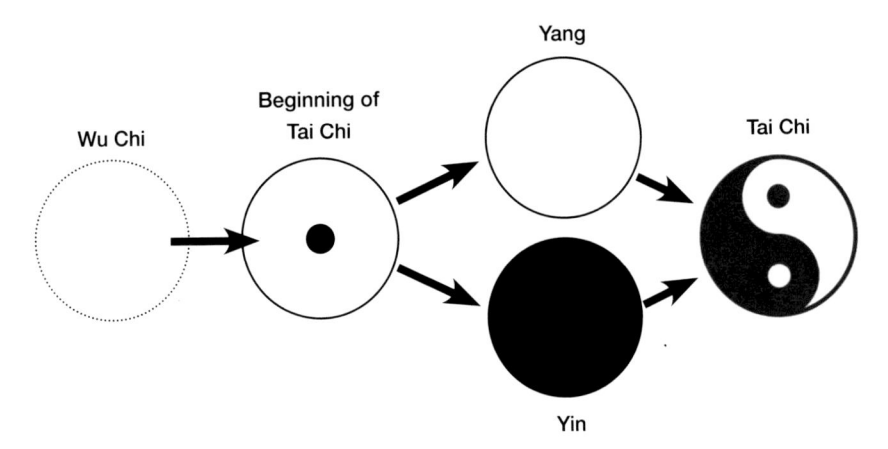

Yin/Yang theory of the origins of the universe

  For Tai Chi practice, I think it's helpful to think of this idea of Yin and Yang not so much as being individual elements in opposition to each other or as existing entirely on their own, but as complements of each other. They unite to form a whole. Although they may be opposite in nature, there is an interdependence between them. Nothing is absolutely Yin or Yang.

  Besides describing their belief in the origins of the universe, the philosophers used Yin-Yang to also describe the relationships between all living and inanimate things in the world. Night or darkness would be an example of Yin, daytime or light an example of Yang; Earth would be an example of Yin, sky an example of Yang; female would be an example of Yin, male an example of Yang. Soft and hard, empty and full, water and fire, south and north, winter and summer—they are all separate entities, yet they only exist with each other. Even the body's vital organs are described as Yin and Yang. The heart, liver, spleen, lung and kidneys are Yin organs, those that filter or transfer/convert energy. The small and large intestines, stomach, gall bladder, bladder, and pericardia are considered Yang organs, ones that either take in nutrients or expel them. (See the Targeting chapter for information about working with your vital organs.)

The concept of Yin and Yang has a direct correlation to practicing Tai Chi. The practice of Tai Chi is an attempt to bring a number of varying, opposite elements into a complementary whole. Simple stepping is a Yin and Yang movement—raising the foot off the floor and then placing it down. The principal of softness and hardness is well captured in the words from the classic Tai Chi writings describing the body as "a steel bar wrapped in cotton" achieving inner strength without external, muscular tension. Stepping can be done softly and gracefully while maintaining a rock-solid stance.

The various postures in the form are also balanced, represented by mirror images of one another. Often when you do a series of movements to the right side, the same series of movements will be duplicated to the left side in another part of the form. Similarly with rising and sinking in the stances, and with movements where you balance on just the right leg and then later on just the left leg, the concept of Yin and Yang, or being well-balanced, is fundamental.

We have discussed in length elsewhere in the book the importance of having balanced breathing. The inhale portion of the breath is considered Yin and the exhale is considered Yang. You optimally want to have the same volume of air on the inhale as you do the exhale. You also want the length of time of your inhale to be identical to the length of time of your exhale. Achieving unity, harmony, and balance with your breath is essential.

Yin and Yang also represent *change*. When one facet weakens, the other strengthens to balance the whole. Yin and Yang elements are always balancing and rebalancing toward a state of harmony and equilibrium. This change is especially apparent in the way the body moves in the Tai Chi form, when weight is transferred, when balancing on one leg, or turning, rising and sinking. The correct shift in Yin and Yang helps maintain our equilibrium. This also allows for the pace of movement to be done slowly without any abrupt movements, or sudden speeding up or slowing down. The great variety of balanced positions in which the body is placed throughout the form creates an almost 360-degree, spherical circulation of Chi when done properly.

By balancing and bringing together all these elements, the original philosophers and those who have practiced it since, have all had a goal of achieving good health. When this balance is compromised, then illness, anxiety, pain, and other negative outcomes can occur. Achieving this balance has also been my emphasis throughout this book.

San Pao

Another important concept in Chi Kung practice is San Pao or "The Three Treasures." San Pao (pronounced "San Pow") refers to the bringing together of three elements called Jing, Chi and Shen. Jing (pronounced "Ching") means our "essence;" Chi is our "internal energy;" and Shen (pronounced "Sun") is one's spirit. Once again, unifying or bringing into harmony individual elements is the key in getting the most out of an internal training practice. The classic writings on the subject say that one needs to "firm the Jing, convert it to Chi, and then nourish the Shen."

The word Jing can mean several things in Chinese, and be both a noun and a verb, but for our purposes, Jing refers to our most primal substance that gives us life. Once you are born, it is the root of your life, given to you by your parents. Jing is stored in the kidneys. Through the concentrated and controlled breathing techniques done in Tai Chi and other Chi Kung exercises, we "firm" or "refine" our Jing, building it up and converting it to Chi that is then stored in our Tan Tien. This is much like opening an IRA savings account, working with and building its value so we can later convert it to cash when needed.

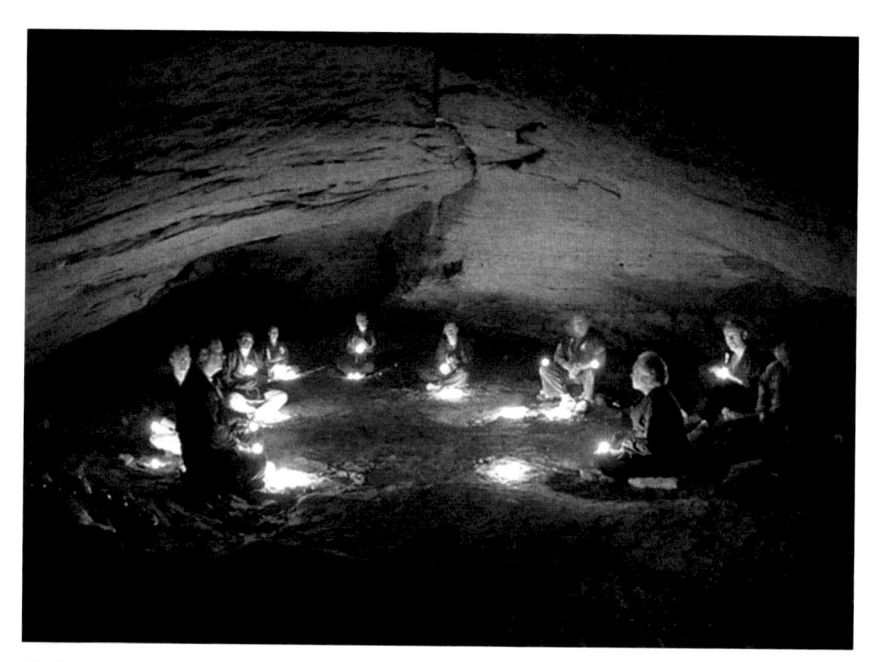

Meditation cave, Furnace Mountain, Kentucky

The Chi then acts as a fuel or sustenance to nourish the Shen. By feeding with Chi, you cultivate or "raise the Shen." The Shen is directed by the mind—a control center of sorts—using the Yie as its CPU or brain to operate the system. The more efficiently the Chi is supplied to the Shen, the more elevated the Shen becomes. The more elevated the Shen, the more your senses are heightened and your mind becomes sharper and more inspired. The ultimate goal of the Three Treasures is to balance the entire system of Jing, Chi and Shen in order to bring oneself to a much higher level of health and longevity.

As with some of the other philosophical subjects that we have touched on in this chapter, there is a depth of information and study about it that is well beyond the scope of this book. Please seek out the wealth of information available elsewhere for a greater understanding.

Because the use of the mind is so important in Chi Kung, we want to also develop a harmony of Hsin and Yie in our general make-up for the most balanced state of mind.

Philosophy & Foundation

Mental Training

As I have pointed out, the best overall health is achieved by unifying the mind, body, and spirit. Our physical, mental, and emotional sides are ultimately not separated and work as "one" when practicing Tai Chi. In today's world, however, many people suffer from problems related to mental stresses and other cognitive issues. Their lives get out of balance. Many seek ways to numb the stresses with illegal and prescription drugs, alcohol, repression, or extreme and dangerous behavior. I think it is well worth mentioning how we can be productive in addressing these problems with Tai Chi training.

Obviously, Tai Chi's goals of achieving a calm and peaceful state, releasing tension, and "letting go" are examples of ways to attain better mental health. Ridding the mind of the noise and negative thoughts, overcoming outside distractions, and gaining an accurate view of ourselves are all results of productive Tai Chi practice. But Tai Chi practice also embodies the same characteristics essential to any kind of human success and personal satisfaction: innovation, flexibility, creativity, motivation, endurance, self-discipline, and expanded personal awareness. Tai Chi uses both the right and left sides of our brain—our imagination and our logic. The effort alone that it takes to practice regularly helps build a disciplined and strong makeup.

Many people have the impression that the meditative arts are only for hermits who ponder alone on a mountain. But they can offer so much to all of us. Regular Tai Chi practice allows us to live life fully. It teaches us to be an active participant in life's joys as well as its challenges.

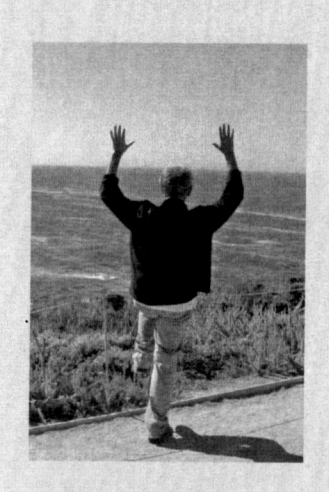

> *When something is earned through time, patience, and effort, it resides in you—you own it. The effort of self-study, searching, and self-cultivation is, I think, the pursuit of a better understanding of the meaning of our lives.*

CHI KUNG & EFFORT

Chi Kung is the science of cultivating the body's life force or Chi. Translated as "Energy Work," Chi Kung practice has roots that go back in China at least 4000 years. The practice is based on the theory of Yin and Yang which describes the relationship of complementary qualities such as soft and hard, female and male, dark and light, or slow and fast, for example. According to this theory, nature tries to harmonize these qualities for balance. For us, achieving that balance can result in improved health, greater self-awareness, and overall fitness.

The concept of Chi is the foundation of traditional Chinese medical theory and Chi Kung. Like the Greek "pneuma" and the Indian Sanskrit "prana," Chi is considered to be the vital force and energy flow in all living things, circulating through channels in the body. Chi Kung theory says when this Chi flow becomes stagnant or stops, illness, pain, or mental and emotional problems occur. Chi Kung practice seeks to not only increase the level of Chi, but restore and improve its circulation. Acupuncture is also based on this theory.

Philosophy & Foundation

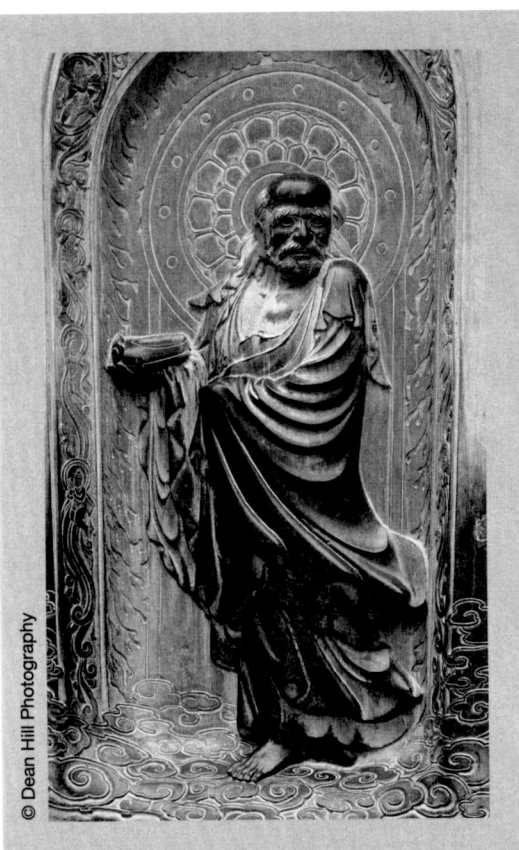

Most researchers credit an Indian monk, Da Mo, also known as Bodhidharma, with not only founding the Chan (Zen) sect of Buddhism, but with becoming the father of Chinese martial arts by incorporating Chi Kung practice into sets of exercises at the original Shaolin temple in Henan province around 550 A.D. The monks at the temple practiced these methods and found that they greatly improved not only their health, but increased their strength and power. The Shaolin monks further developed these techniques by integrating them with sets of martial arts forms that imitated the movements of animals known for their fighting prowess, like the tiger, dragon, praying mantis, snake, and crane. Later and outside the temple, other meditative martial arts practices that use Chi training, like Tai Chi Chuan and Pa Kua Chang, were developed

Our present day Chung Yen Shaolin martial arts group often refers to the practice of Chi Kung as "internal" or Nei Kung. Not only does it include more typical still-type meditation and focused breathing, but also incorporates the use of Chi Kung techniques with stances, punches, kicks, sparring, conditioning and endurance training. Our regular martial arts classes usually starting incorporating Nei Kung at the intermediate level and add more complex material at advanced levels.

Like our Lee Family Tai Chi classes, we also offer Chi Kung classes for both martial arts and non-martial arts students. We use some or all of Bodhidharma's original 18 position set of exercises to help with the practice. Through concentration and special breathing techniques, we first help students accumulate and increase their Chi. We then help train them to mentally focus on their breath and at the same time, imagine guiding energy to their vital organs and throughout the body while maintaining several different body postures. The postures and techniques are actually not very complicated and can be quickly learned with the proper guidance. It is one's regular effort, focus, and diligence in the practice of these techniques that brings the benefits. Think of this equation: Greater Effort + Increased Time + Volume = More Efficiency.

One of the greatest benefits of Chi Kung practice is what is earned *through the effort that it takes* rather than something attained. The "Kung" in Chi Kung is the same as in "Kung Fu," which is a term often used to refer to Chinese martial arts, but is literally translated "energy-time." Some attainment is like inherited wealth; obtained without effort or discipline. As a result, it is soon depleted or loses its value. When something is earned through time, patience, and effort, it resides in you—you own it. The effort of self-study, searching, and self-cultivation is, I think, the pursuit of a better understanding of the meaning of our lives.
—*David Cubine*

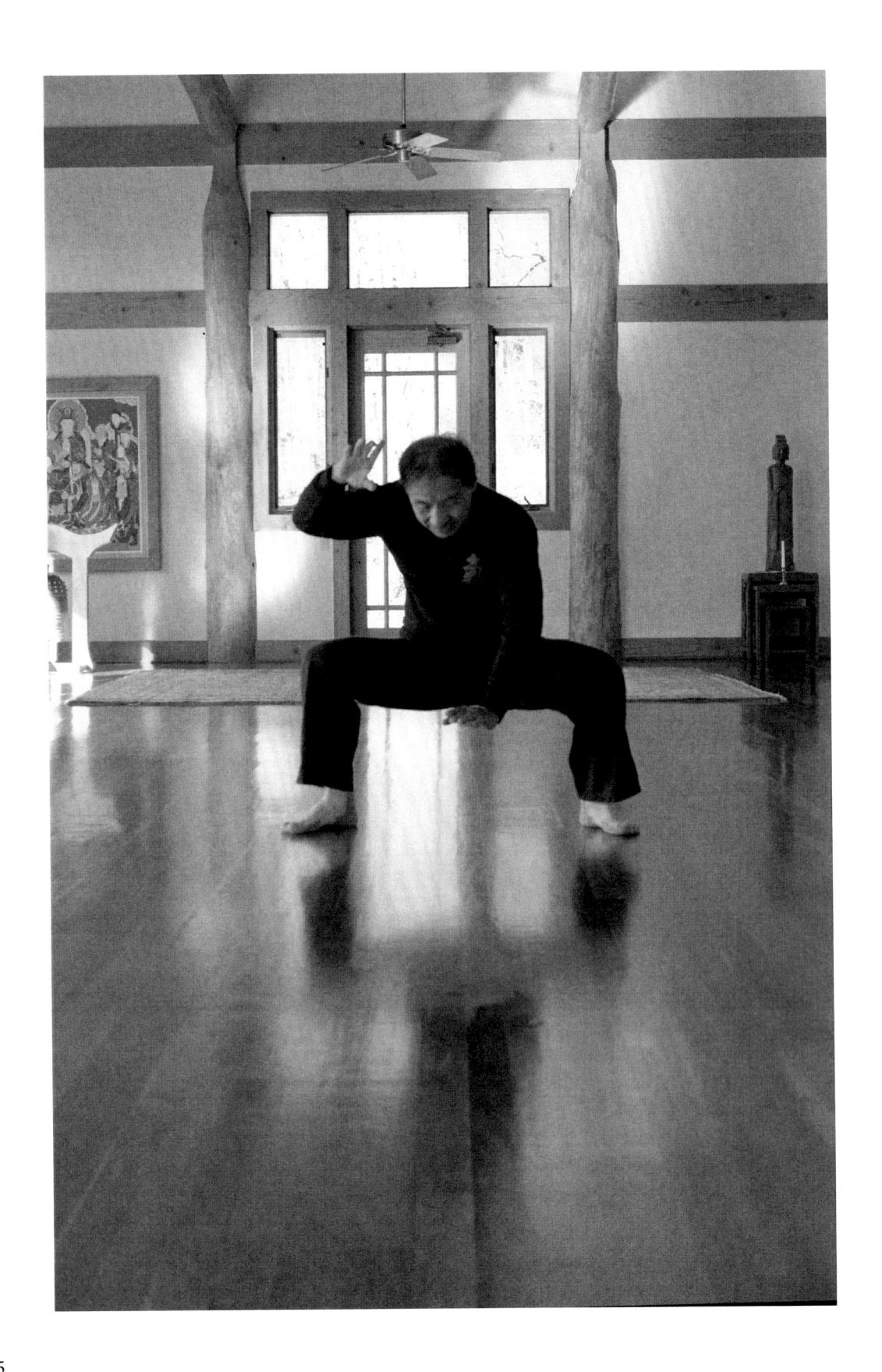

FIVE

LEE CHIA TAI CHI CHUAN: THE FORM

THIS CHAPTER PRESENTS PHOTOS AND DESCRIPTIVE TEXT for each of the Lee Family Tai Chi Chuan's 60 postures. The photos and text are a supplement to the companion DVD which includes both the complete form and the form broken down into smaller sections. The book's Form chapter and the video each have their own advantages—the photos can be used to clearly identify the hand, arm, leg, and body positions for each posture, while the video better demonstrates how the postures are connected, and the speed, pace, and the timing of the movements.

For each posture, the photos present a front view and a side view showing the inhale movement and then the exhale movement. Each view has an arrow pointing "east," the direction faced at the start of the form, to help identify the correct orientation. Each posture also contains a symbol of the vital organ or meridian associated with that posture. For a complete list of each posture and the associated vital organ or meridian, see appendix A.

In our Beginner Lee Family Tai Chi classes, we teach an average of five postures per class over a 12-week course. You can follow the individual sections of the video to closely match the class schedule. As with the in-person classes, we recommend that students spend some time each day practicing the previous section's material before moving on to the next section. And as I tell my in-class students, you will get out of it exactly what you put into it—if you spend some time practicing on your own, I know *you will be rewarded*. It's that simple.

I would like to bring up a few points about practicing effectively. Sometimes we all want everything yesterday. We become impatient when the stop light doesn't turn green fast enough, when our food order at the restaurant isn't ready quickly enough, or we can't get a packaged delivered overnight. We all have to watch out for that. I urge you to be patient with your learning of Tai Chi and take it one step at a time.

With our hectic lifestyles, we often have to put out a lot of fires. With everything going 100 miles an hour, you don't leave enough time for yourself. Practicing Lee Family Tai Chi Chuan takes only about 12 minutes to do the complete form. I would like you to make those 12 minutes, *quality minutes*—make them *your minutes*.

Another important point is that you should not stress your joints when practicing. You should not feel pain in your ankles, knees, hips, back, neck, elbows, or shoulders. If your posture is incorrect, then your knee, for example, may be overly stressed and hurt. If at any time your joints are in pain, you should try moving your foot position or make other adjustments. We all know that no one's body is exactly the same, so you have to try to let your body tell you what you can do comfortably. Also, you should try to avoid extending your knee beyond the toe of the foot on the same leg. When you do that, you put stress on your knee joint. Sometimes you may think, "I didn't put much pressure on my knee," but you will be surprised how much strain you can apply without realizing it. If for whatever reason, you can't go down as low, or raise your leg as high, or whatever the position, just don't do it. Just back off and then try to improve your performance one step at a time. You can have *productive discomfort*, when your muscles are just sore. That is normally fine. If it's negative pain, either readjust or back off completely.

I also want you to not feel discouraged if you cannot perform all the postures exactly as you see me do them. The deepness of the stances, and the balancing on one leg can be challenging, but you can modify those to match your own comfort level by not going quite as deep in the stances, or by not raising your leg as high when balancing on one leg. I'm confident that, with practice, you will gradually gain more ability over time. See appendix B for a set of specific modifications you can use on several of the more physically challenging postures.

Remember, you are doing Lee Family Tai Chi for your health. Unfortunately, we live in a culture where too many things involve competition, but try to not compare yourself to others or become overly self-conscious when doing Tai Chi. In the end, *just have some fun.*

> **DID YOU KNOW?**
>
> **"So how many moves are in Tai Chi?" The "answer" is....ONE.**
>
> Yes, there are 60 postures, each with an inhale and exhale move, but the feel you want to have when practicing the form is as if you were doing *one continuous* movement. When transitioning from an inhale to an exhale movement, or exhale to inhale movement, you do not come to a complete stop, but the movement is continuous. The end of one posture is actually the beginning of the next posture—there is a slight overlap between the two. Practicing the exercises detailed in the Breathing chapter is a very helpful way to develop this seamless flow and achieve the concept of *one* continuous movement in the Tai Chi form.

Lee Family Tai Chi Chuan is not designed for competition. It's designed for your health...So just have some fun!

POSTURE DESCRIPTION KEY:

RH: Right Hand
LH: Left Hand
RF: Right Foot
LF: Left Foot
CW: Clockwise
CCW: Counter Clockwise
BS: Bo Stance (Weight distribution 60% Front/40% Rear)
HS: Horse Stance (Weight distribution 50%/50%)
CS: Cat Stance (Front leg on ball of foot, weight on back leg. Weight distribution 80% Rear/20% Front)

NOTE: Due to a non-martial arts injury, Hiang Thè's right arm does not fully straighten. On postures where both arms are in similar positions, use the left arm as your reference for the correct position.

Starting Position

Starting Position

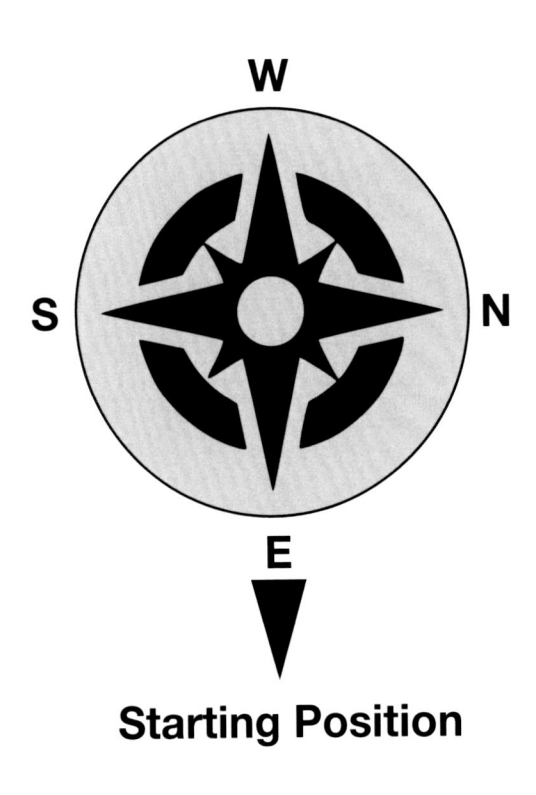

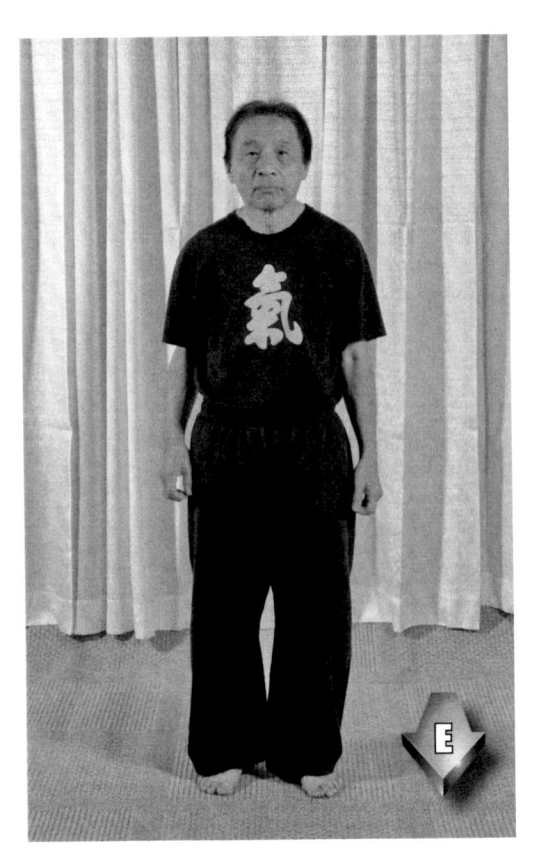

Posture 1

FRONT VIEW

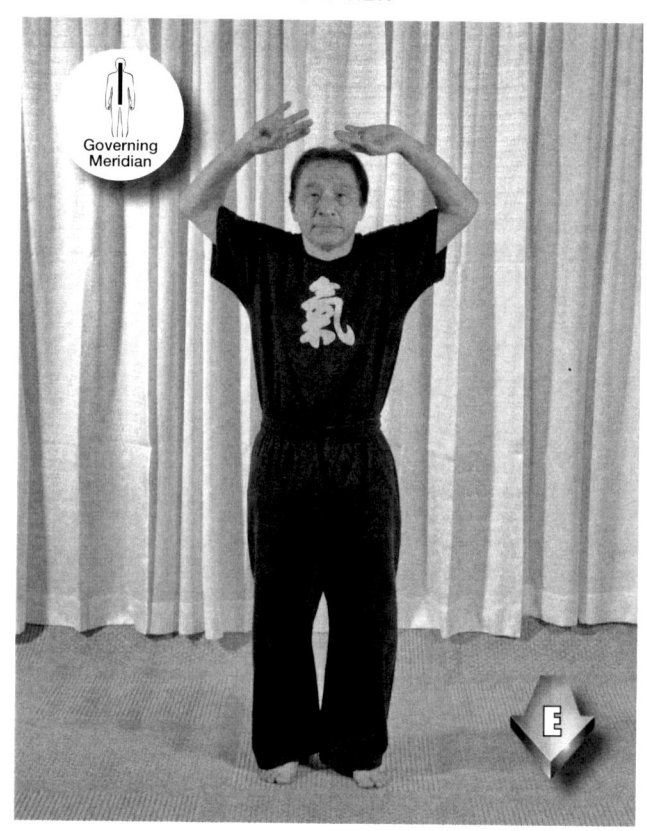

Governing Meridian

SIDE VIEW

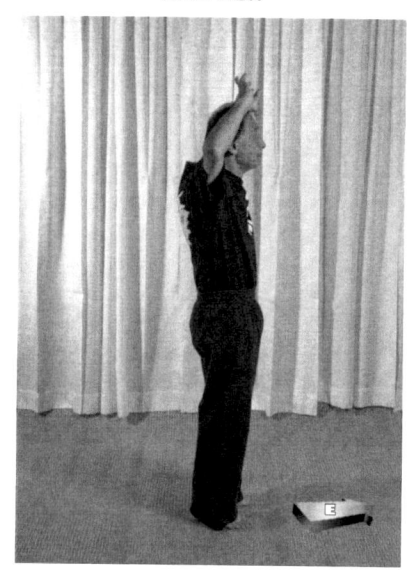

POSTURE 1-*INHALE*
Arms raise out to the sides and up until fingertips point toward each other overhead. End with palms facing upward.

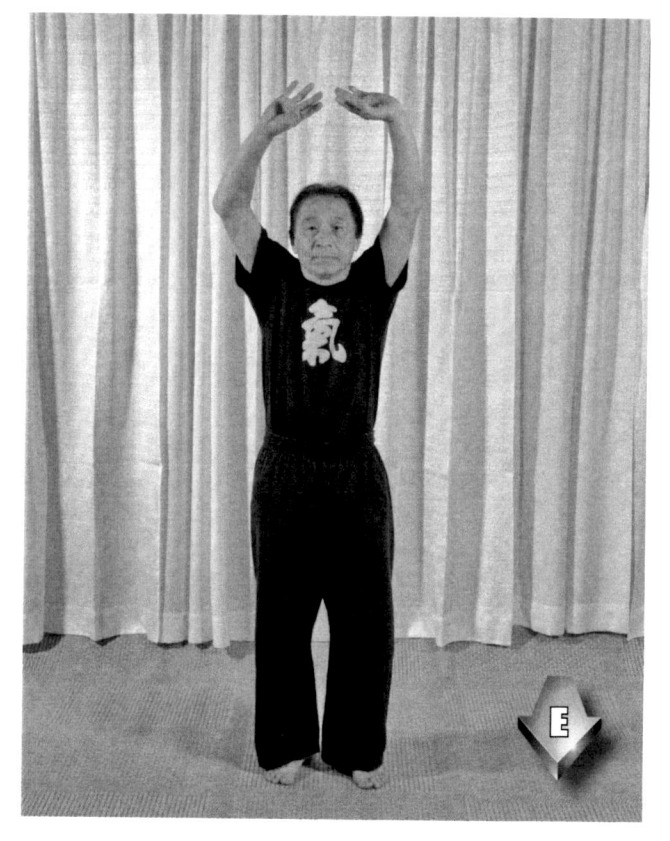

SIDE VIEW

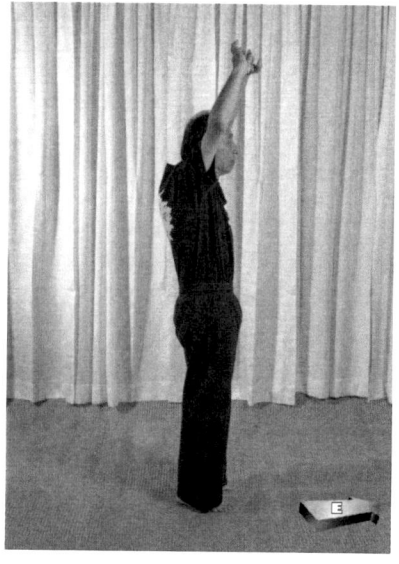

POSTURE 1-*EXHALE*
Extend hands upward.

Posture 2

FRONT VIEW

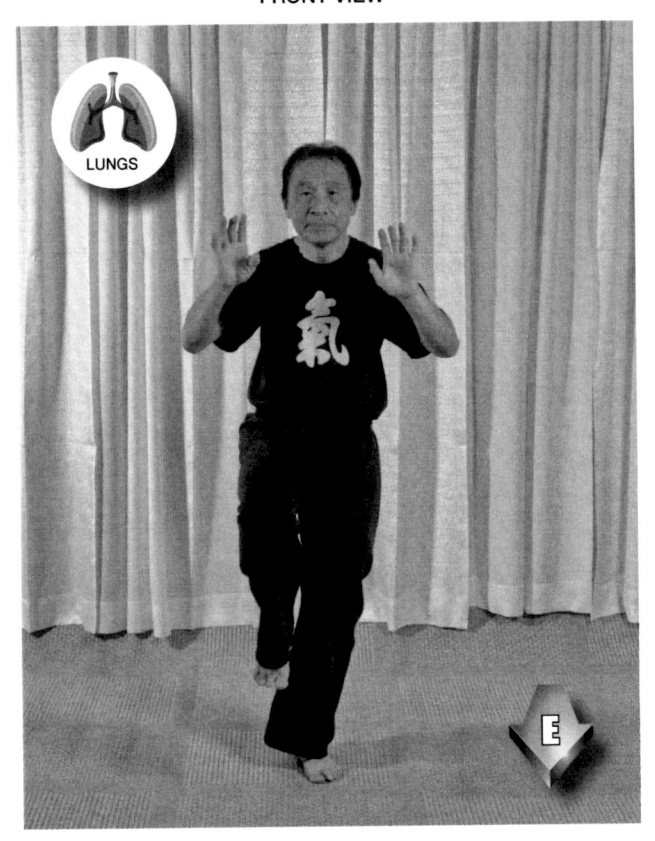

SIDE VIEW

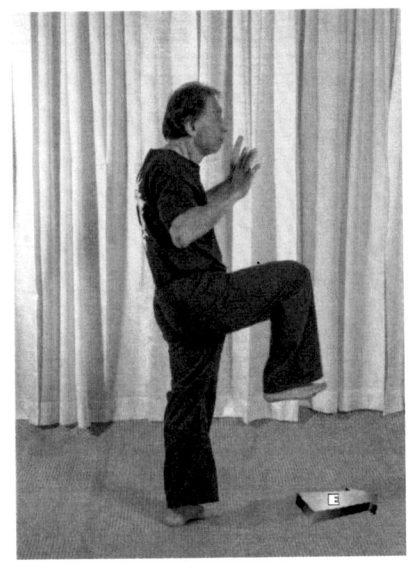

POSTURE 2-*INHALE*
Weight shifts to LF as hands come down to shoulder height with palms facing forward.

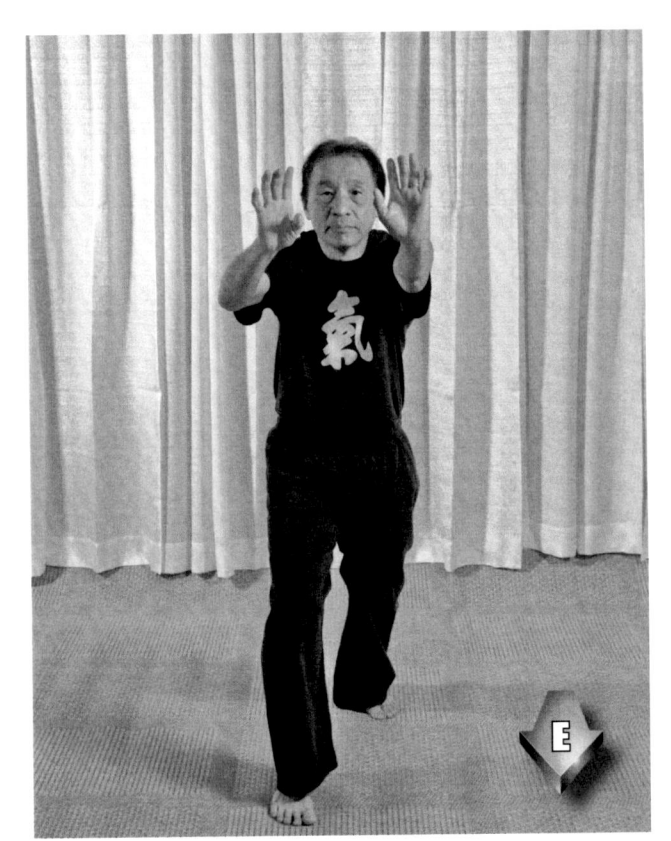

SIDE VIEW

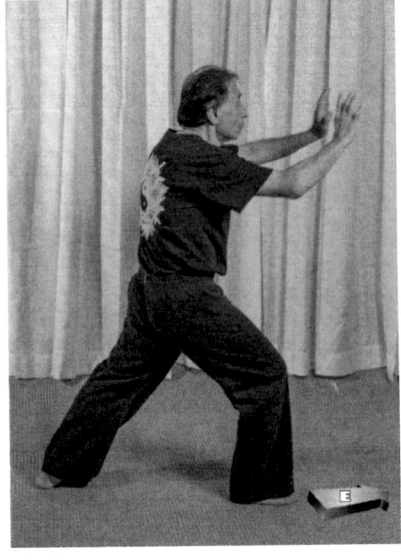

POSTURE 2-*EXHALE*
RF steps forward to BS as hands extend forward, palms facing to the front.

Posture 3

FRONT VIEW

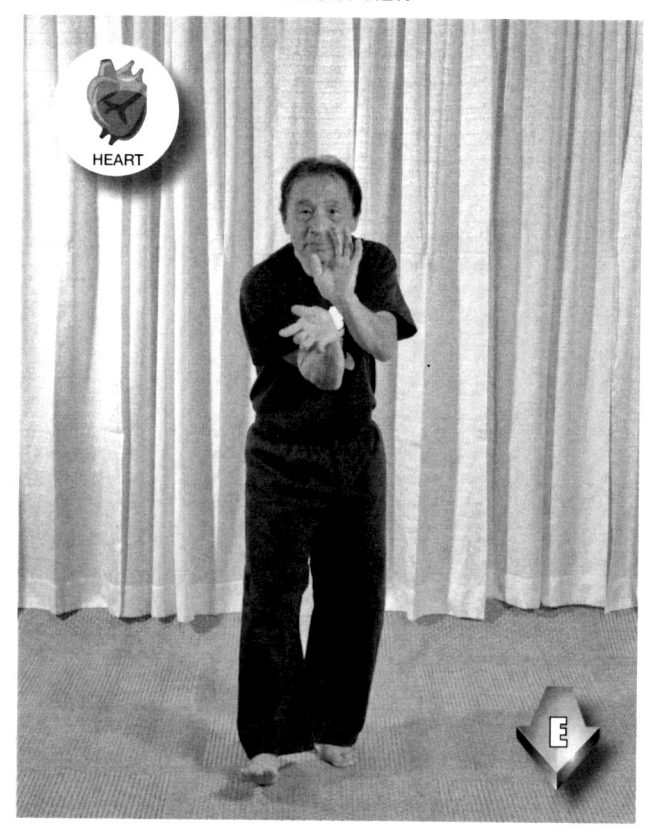

SIDE VIEW

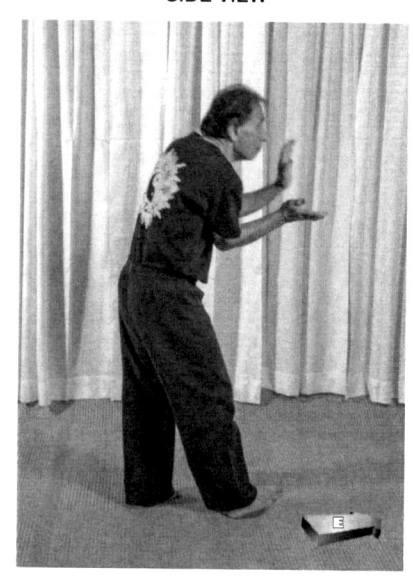

POSTURE 3-*INHALE*
Shift weight to rear leg as RF moves back to heel stance as RH turns 180° CW until fingers are pointing down, both palms facing forward.

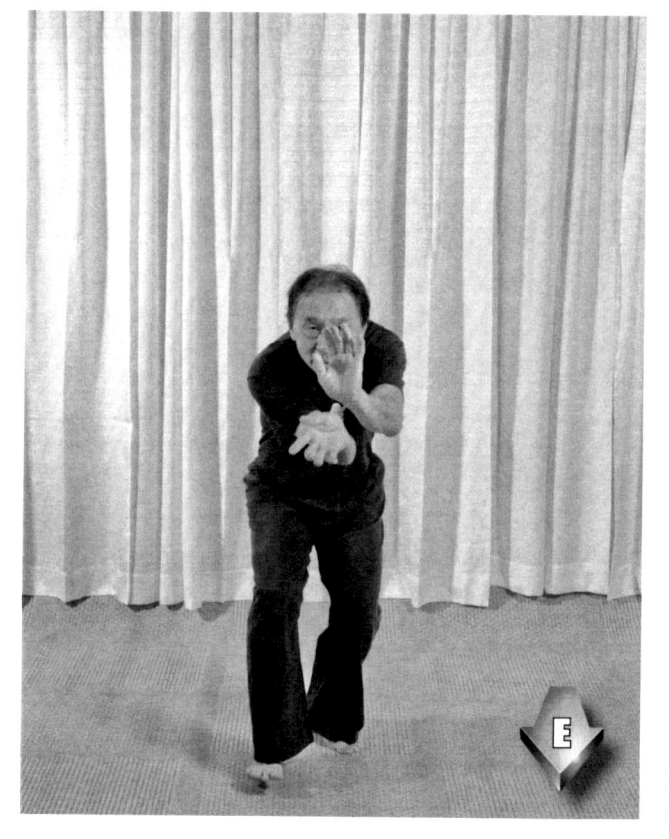

SIDE VIEW

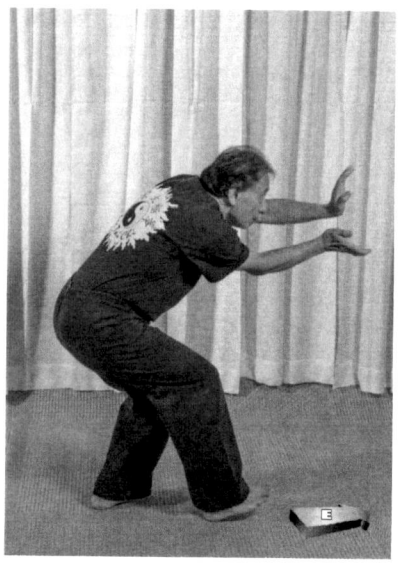

POSTURE 3-*EXHALE*
Sink weight as both hands extend forward.

Posture 4

FRONT VIEW

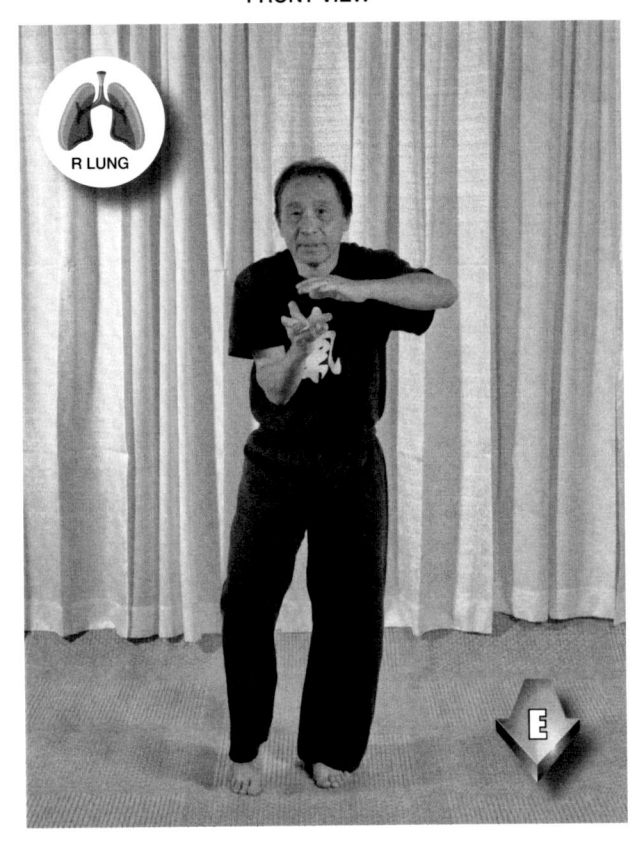

SIDE VIEW

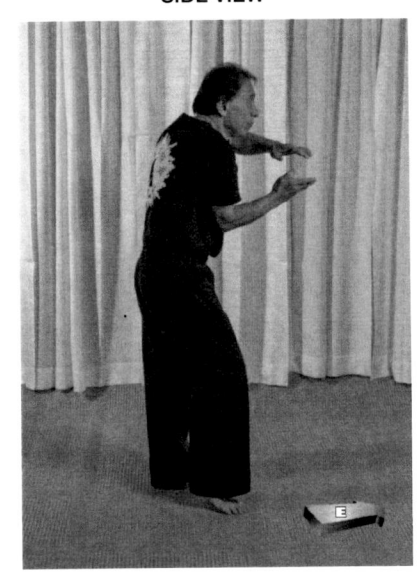

POSTURE 4-*INHALE*
RF shifts to CS as hands come back to chest level in "holding ball" position—palms face each other, LH is on top with fingers pointing to the front, and RH on the bottom with fingers pointing to the left.

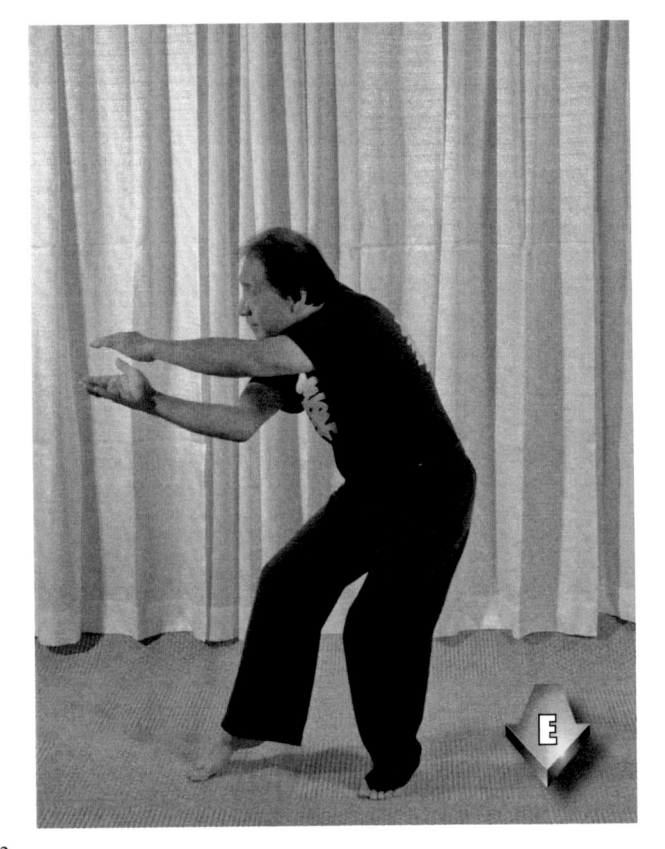

SIDE VIEW

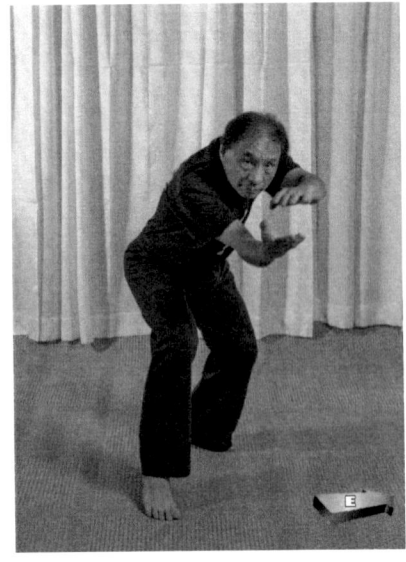

POSTURE 4-*EXHALE*
Body turns 90° to the right, (RF moves before body) as the hands circle to the right with the body, weight staying on LF (Hands still parallel with the floor, palms facing each other)

Posture 5

FRONT VIEW

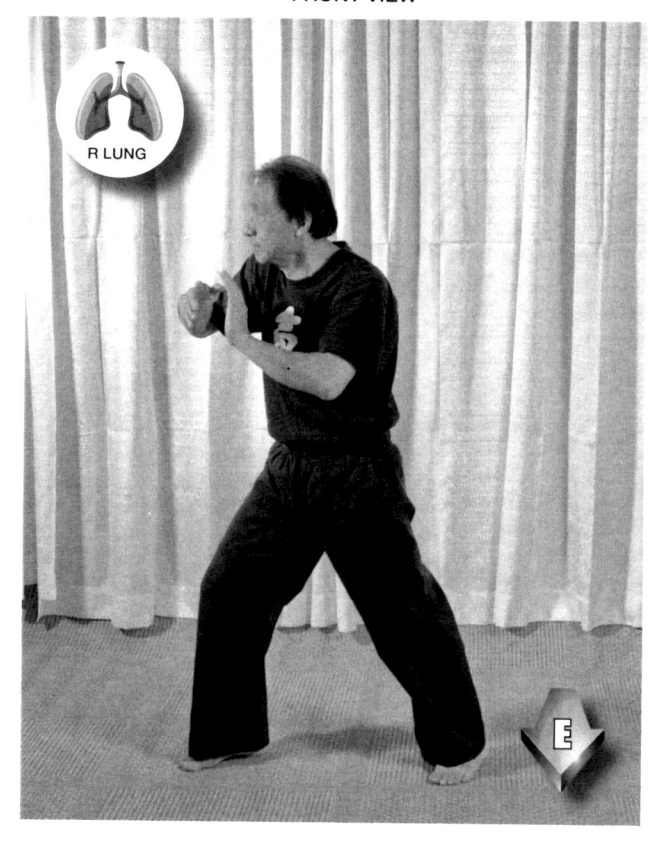

SIDE VIEW

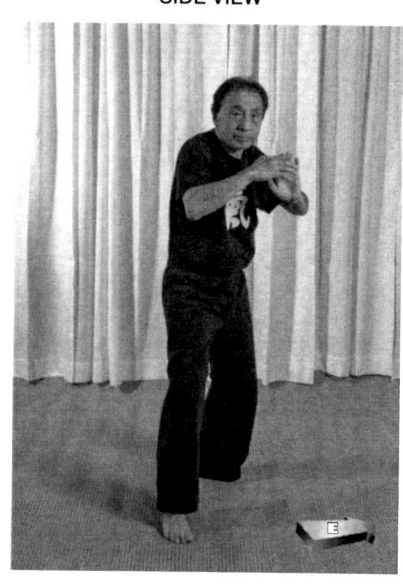

POSTURE 5-_INHALE_
With palms still facing each other, hands rotate so the RH is in the front, fingers to the left, and LH is behind with fingers up. As hands turn, both hands comes back toward the chest.

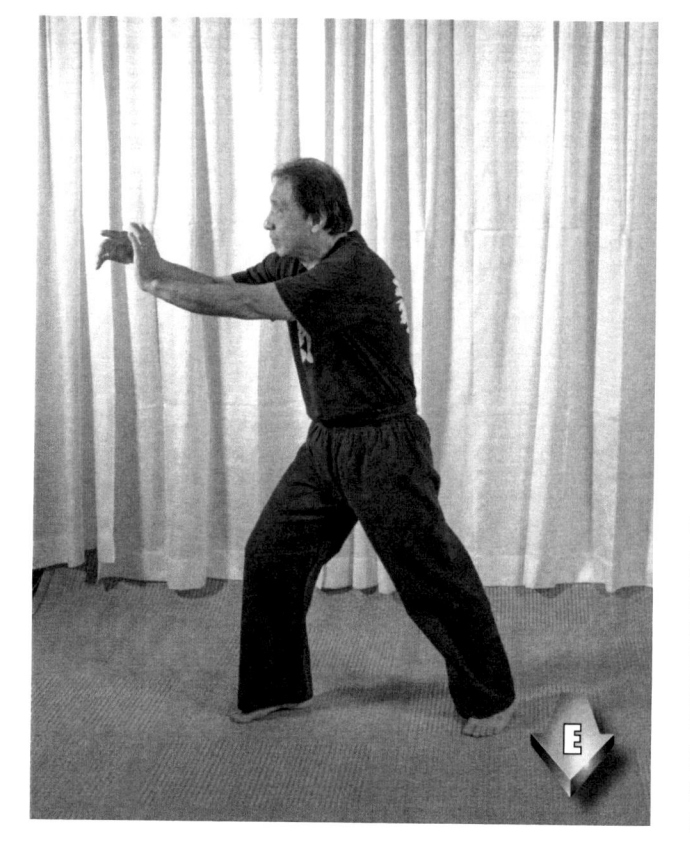

SIDE VIEW

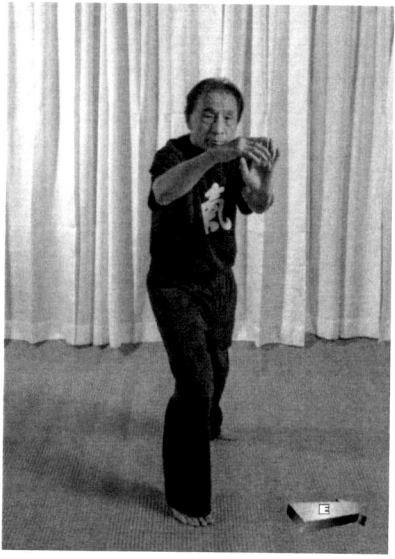

POSTURE 5-_EXHALE_
RF steps to BS as hands extend forward, RH in front.

44

Posture 6

FRONT VIEW

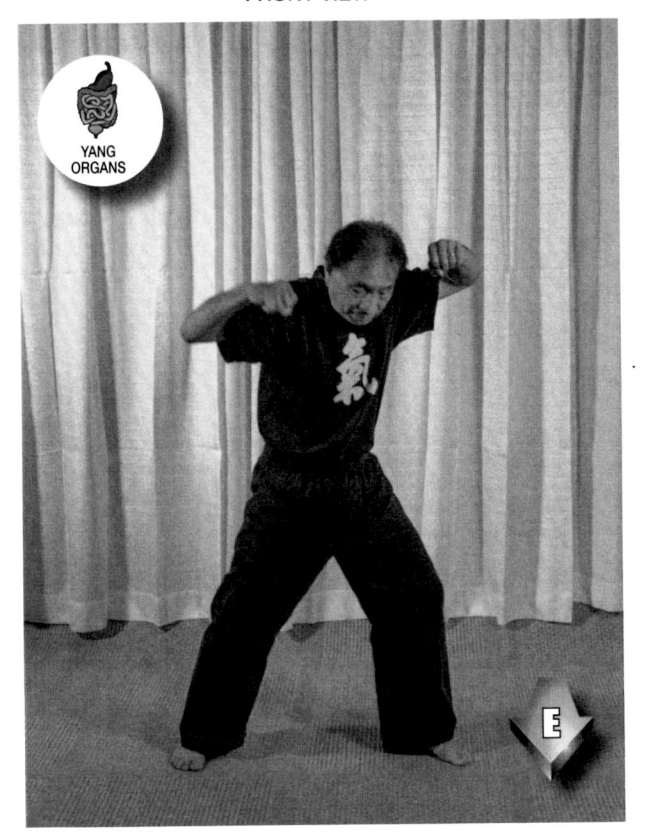

YANG ORGANS

SIDE VIEW

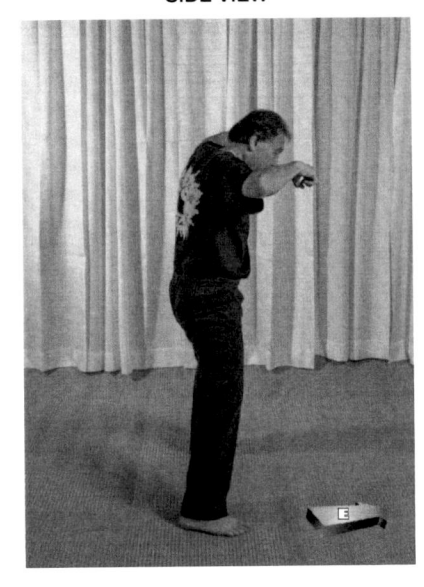

POSTURE 6-*INHALE*
Rotate body 180° to the left as hands pull to above shoulder level. Hands form a loose fist.

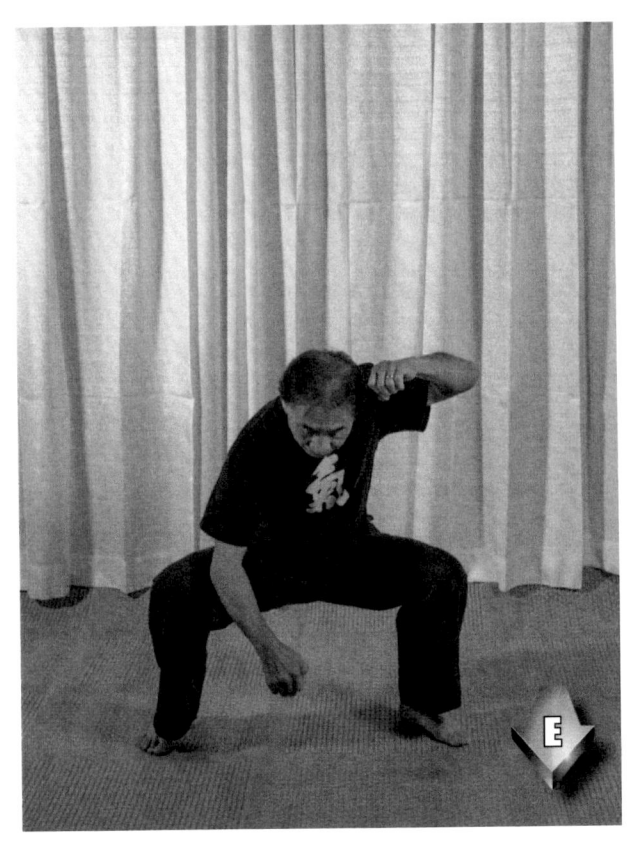

SIDE VIEW

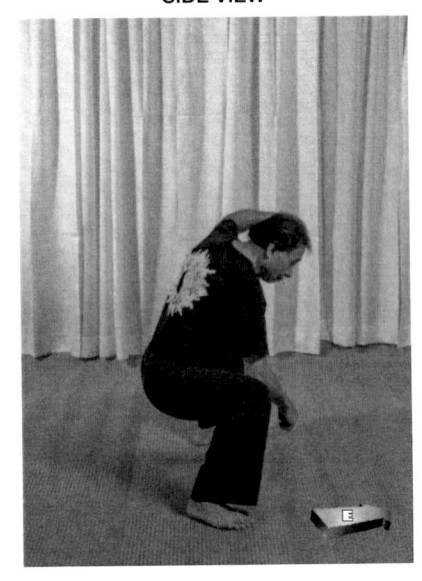

POSTURE 6-*EXHALE*
Right fist extends down to floor between legs. LH remains at left temple. Vision follows right hand.

Posture 7

FRONT VIEW

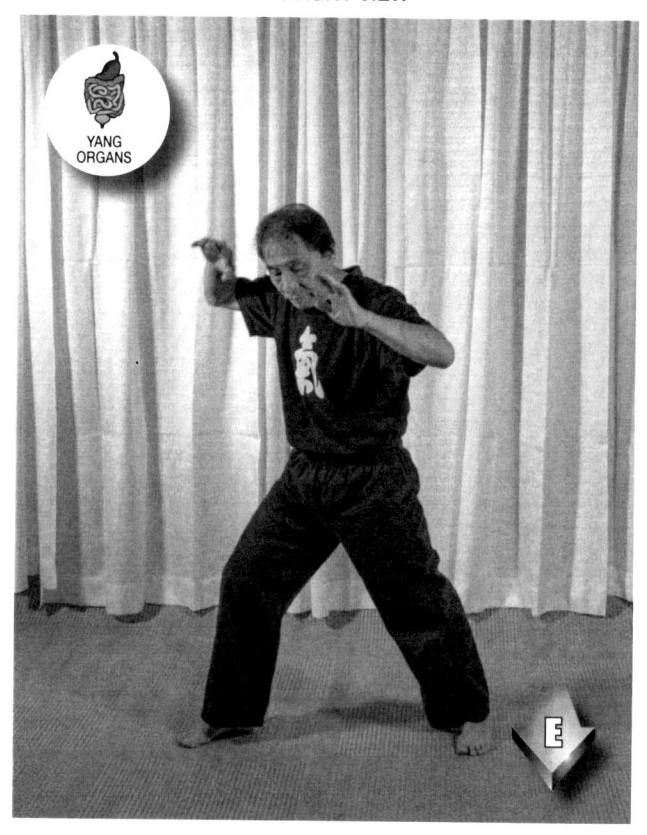

SIDE VIEW

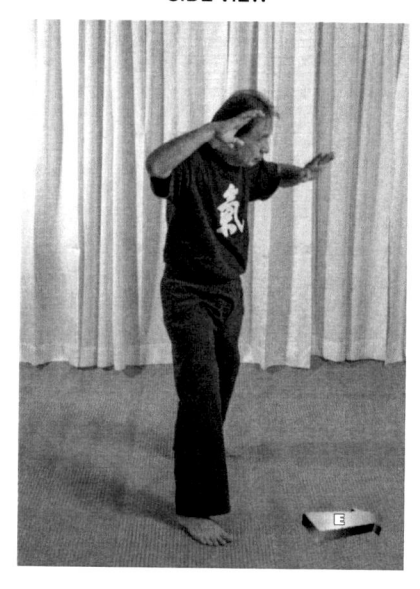

POSTURE 7-*INHALE*
Raise up as body rotates to right, hands open and raise to above shoulder level.

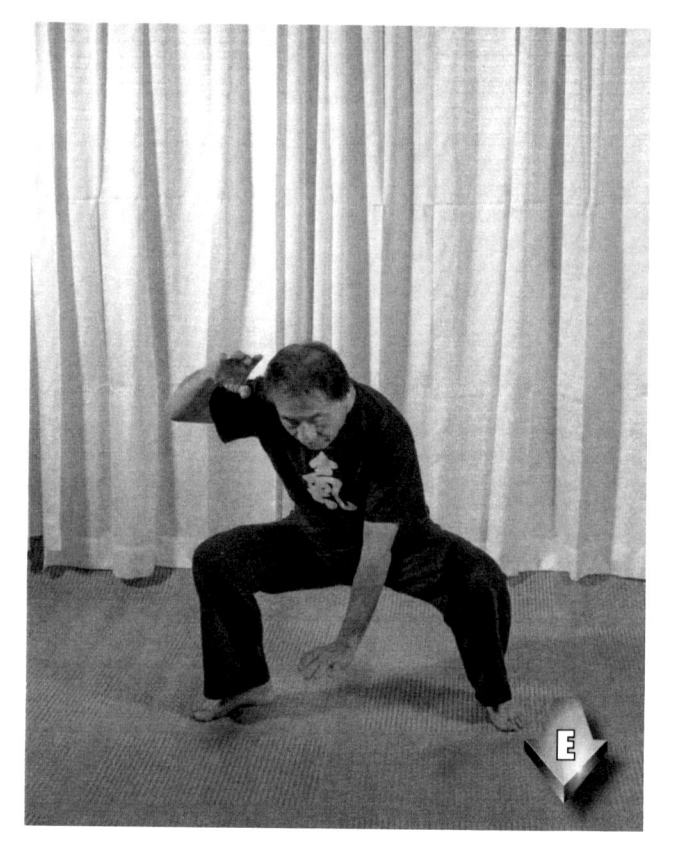

SIDE VIEW

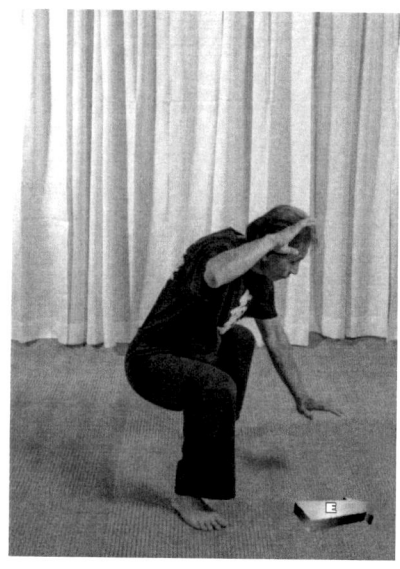

POSTURE 7-*EXHALE*
Both hands are open, as left palm presses down to floor between legs. RH remains at right temple. Vision follows left hand.

Posture 8

FRONT VIEW

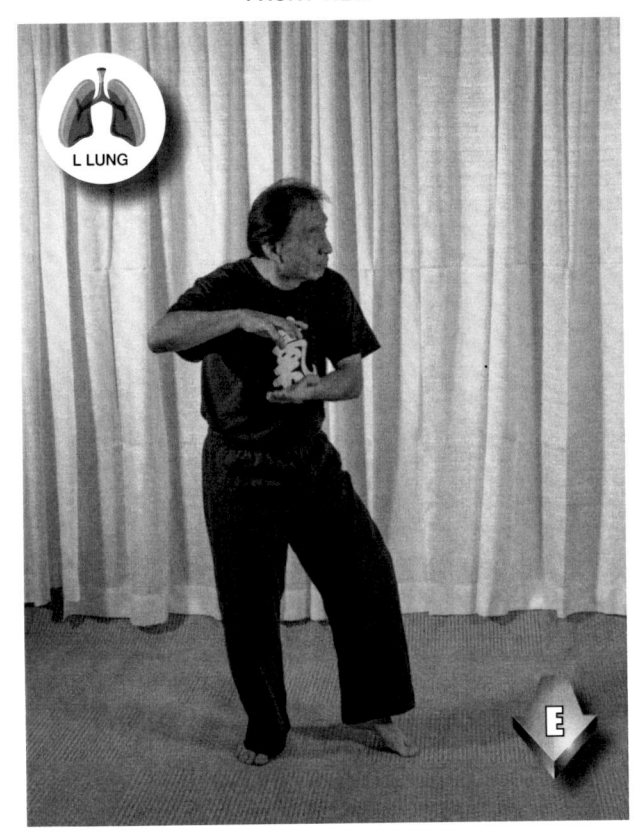

SIDE VIEW

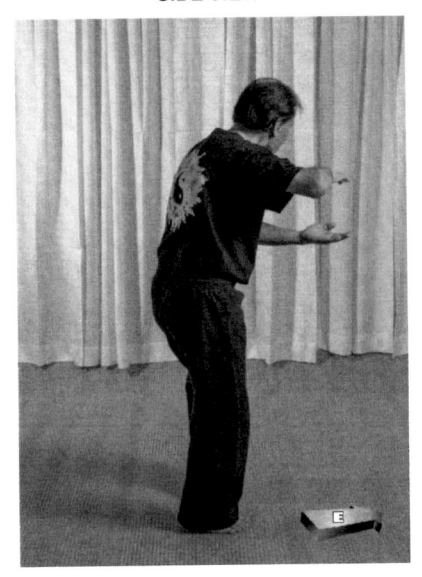

POSTURE 8-*INHALE*
Raise the body, shifting weight to RF and pull LF back to CS. Hands form holding ball position with RH on top.

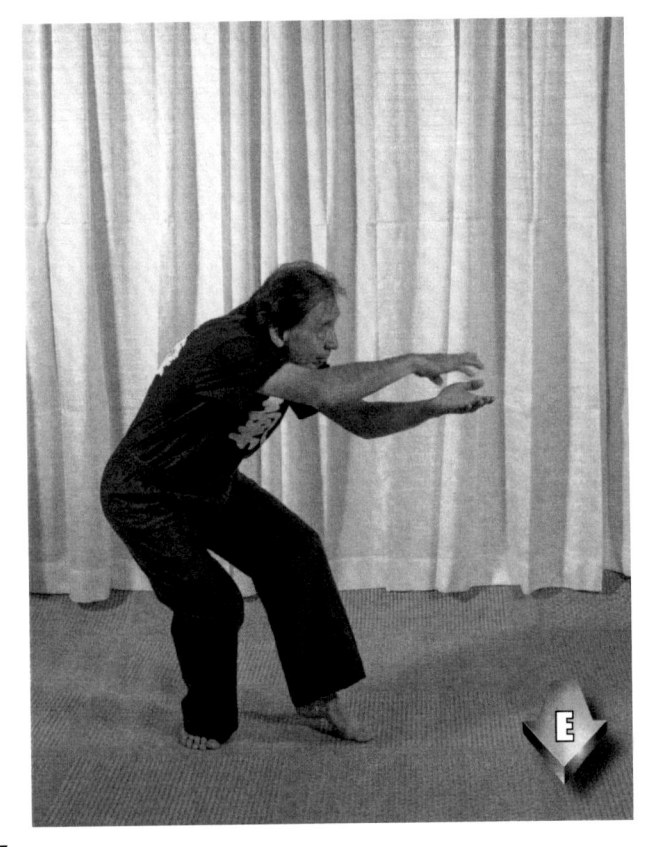

SIDE VIEW

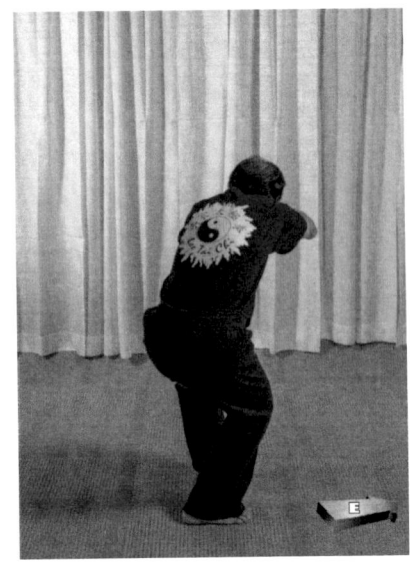

POSTURE 8-*EXHALE*
Hands circle to the left, 80% weight staying on RF (Hands still parallel with the floor, palms facing each other)

Posture 9

FRONT VIEW

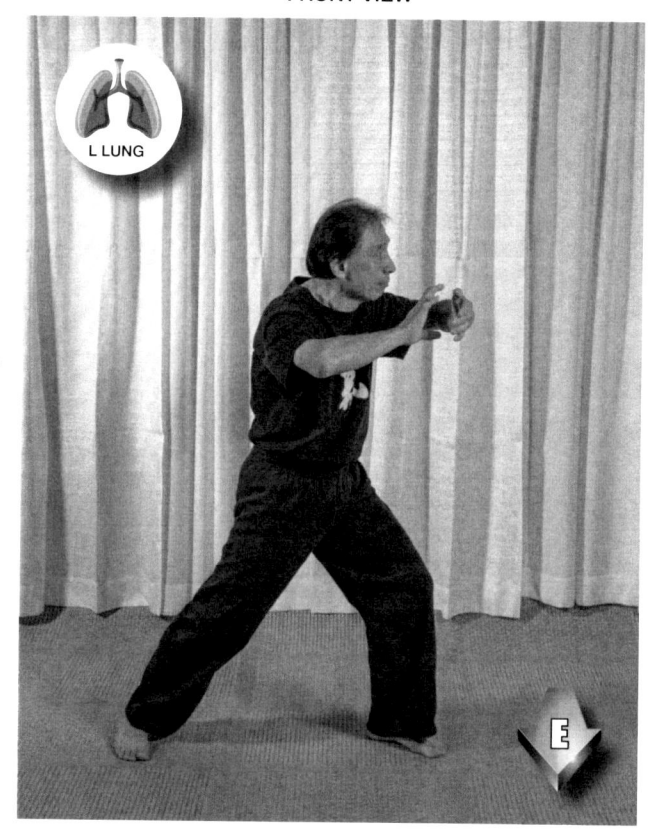

SIDE VIEW

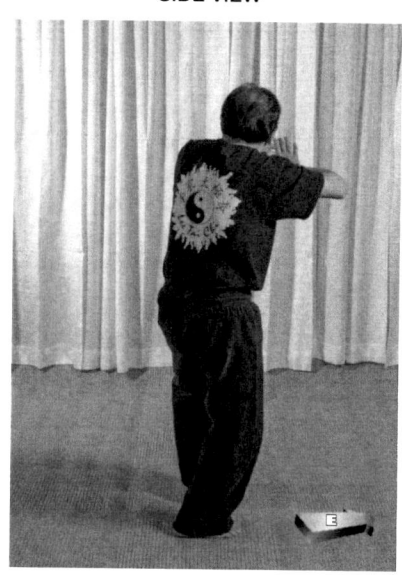

POSTURE 9-_INHALE_
With palms still facing each other, hands rotate so the LH is in the front, fingers pointing to the right, and RH is behind with fingers pointing up. As hands turn, bring both hands back to chest.

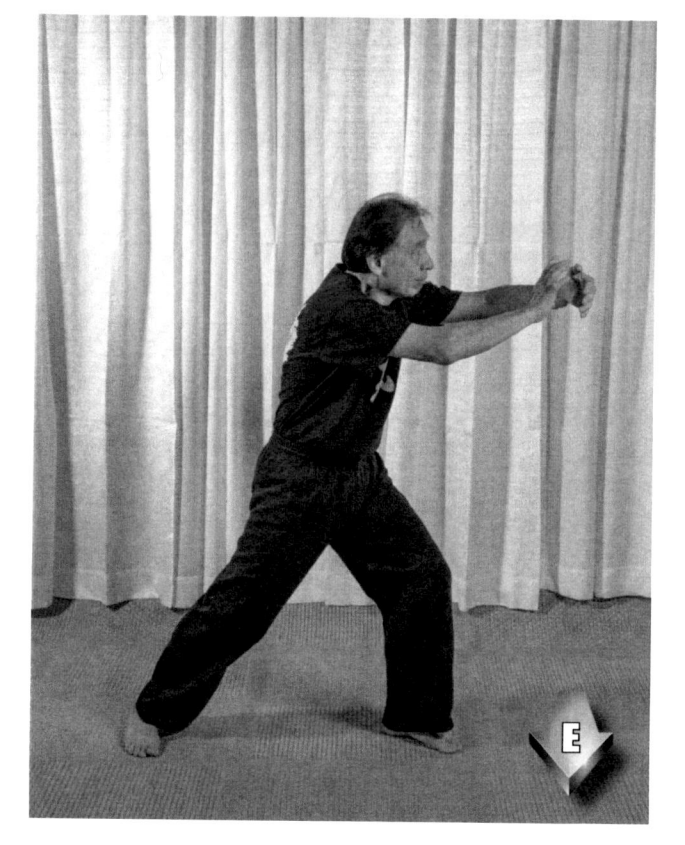

SIDE VIEW

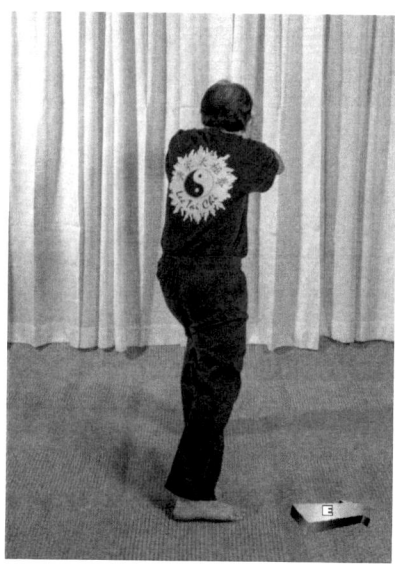

POSTURE 9-_EXHALE_
LF steps to BS as hands extend forward, LH in front.

Posture 10

FRONT VIEW

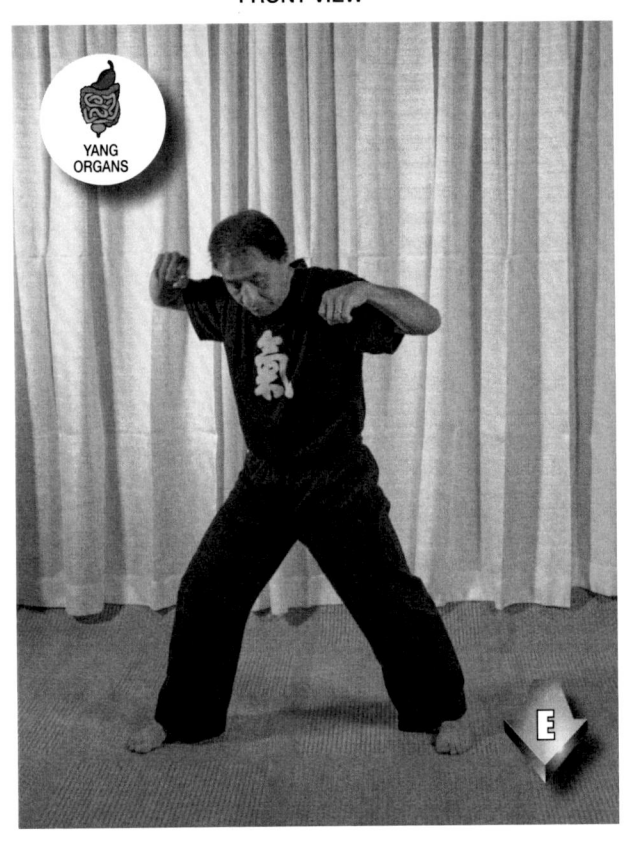

YANG ORGANS

SIDE VIEW

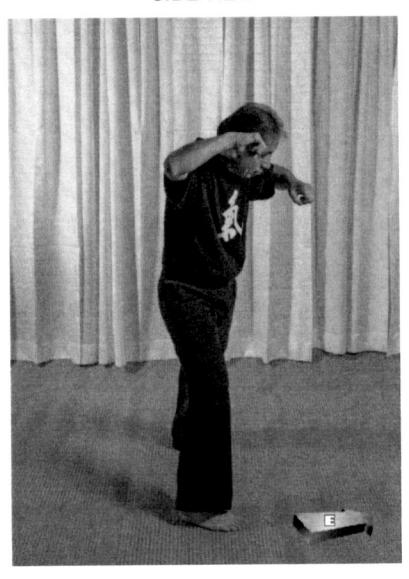

POSTURE 10-*INHALE*
Body rotates 180° to right with hands at above shoulder level in a loose fist.

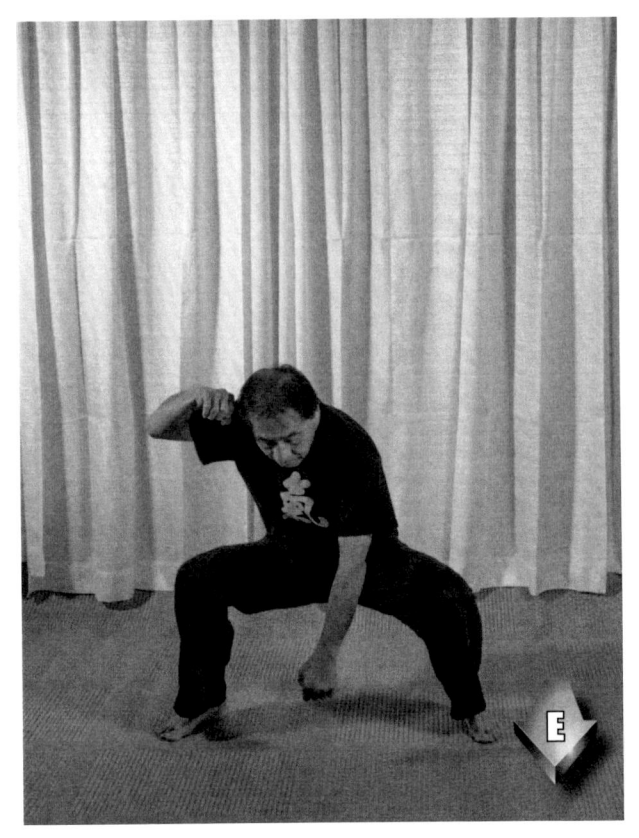

SIDE VIEW

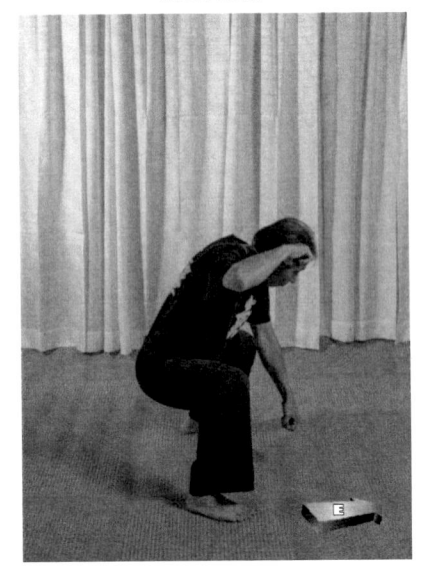

POSTURE 10-*EXHALE*
Left fist presses down to floor between legs. RH at left temple. Vision follows left fist.

Posture 11

FRONT VIEW

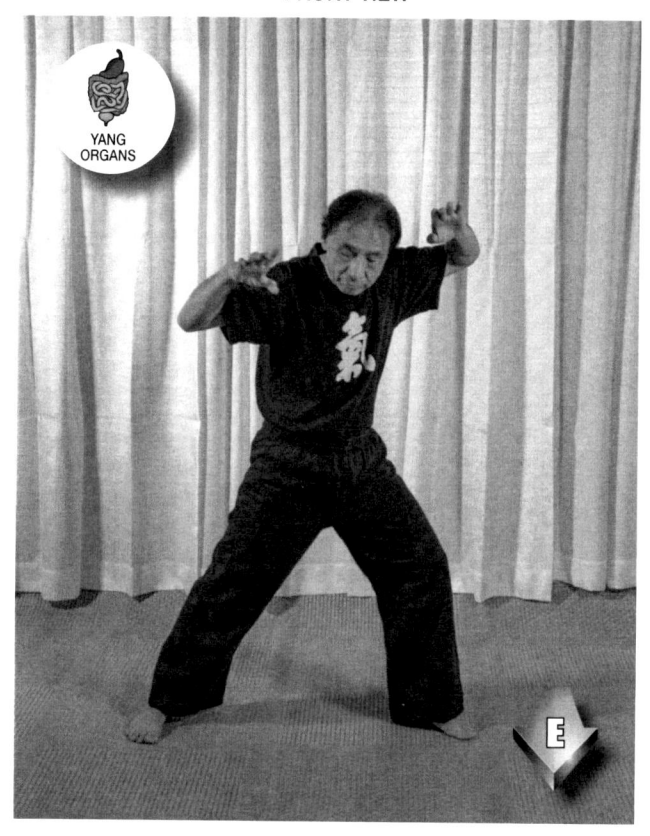

SIDE VIEW

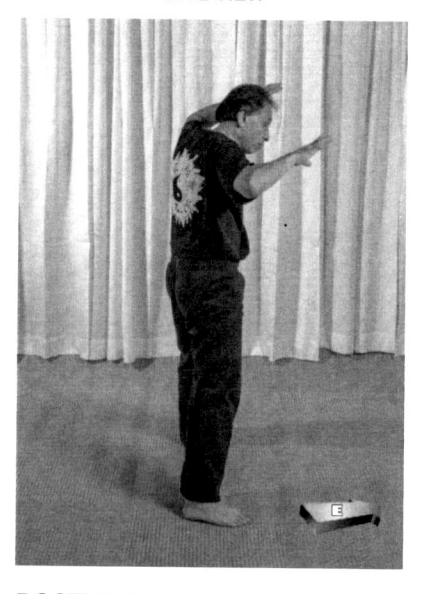

POSTURE 11-*INHALE*
Raise up as body rotates to left with hands open at above shoulder level.

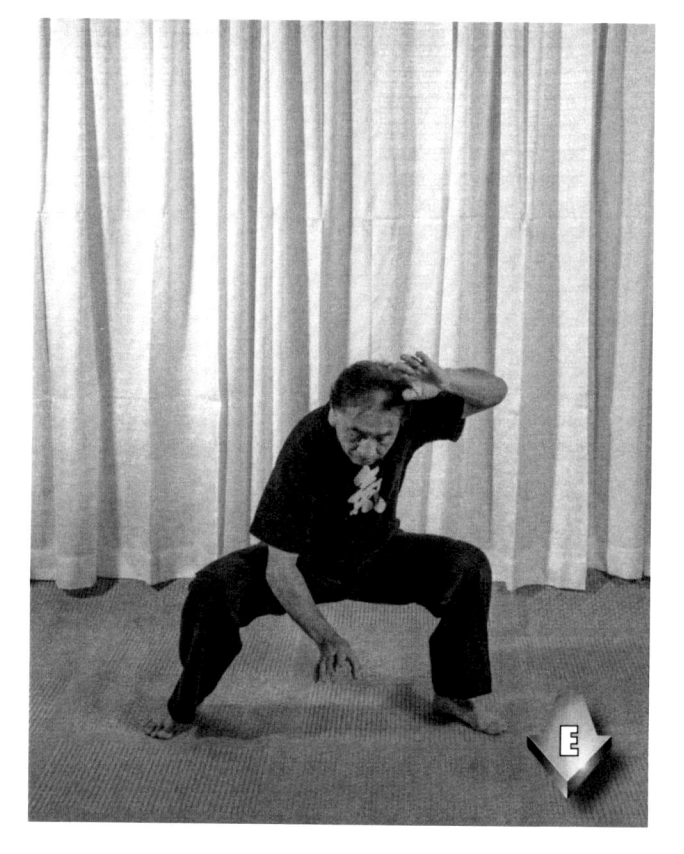

SIDE VIEW

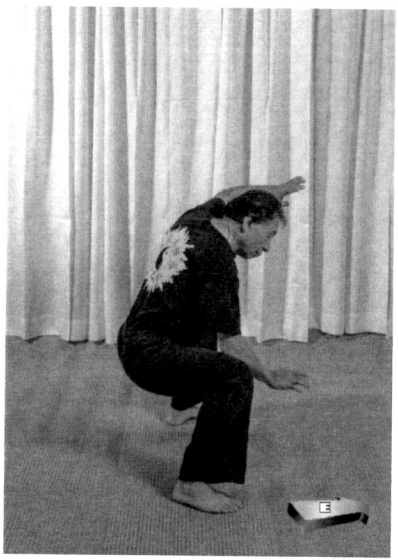

POSTURE 11-*EXHALE*
Right palm presses down to floor between legs. LH is at right temple. Vision follows right hand.

50

Posture 12

FRONT VIEW

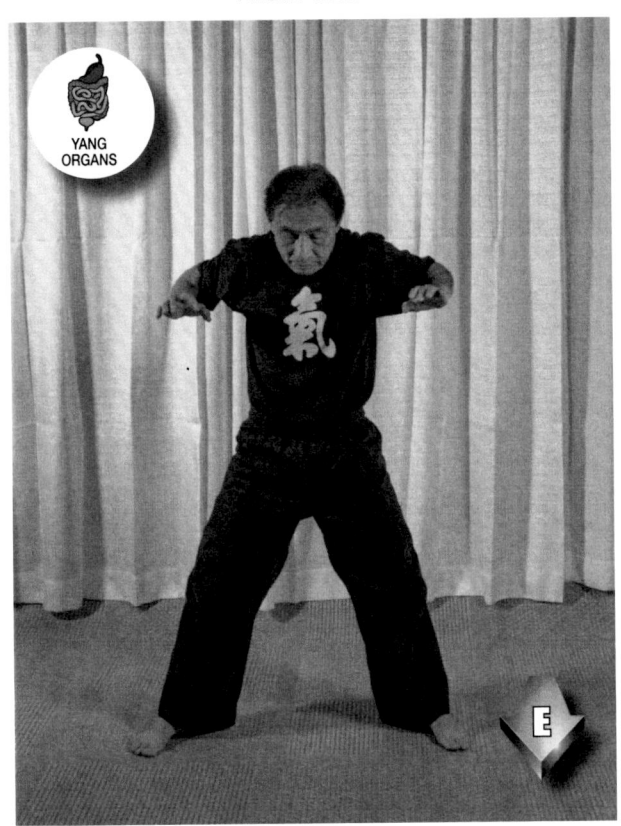

SIDE VIEW

Circle hands sequence

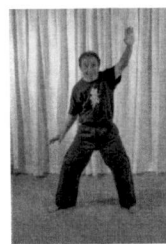

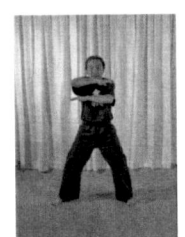

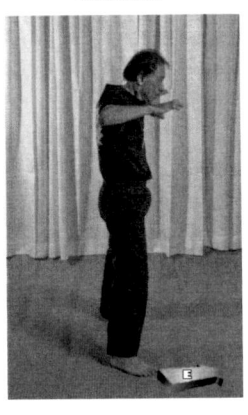

YANG ORGANS

POSTURE
12-*INHALE*
LH extends out to the left as both hands circle in CCW direction and cross in front of body, RH crosses in front. (Body turns facing the front into HS as you circle hands) then both hands pull rearward, palms down, as you expand the chest.

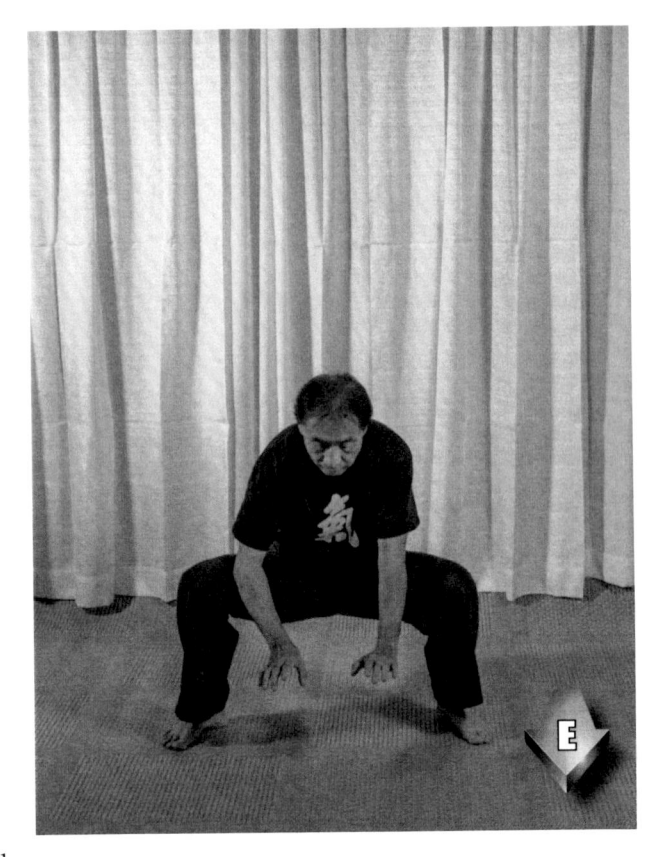

SIDE VIEW

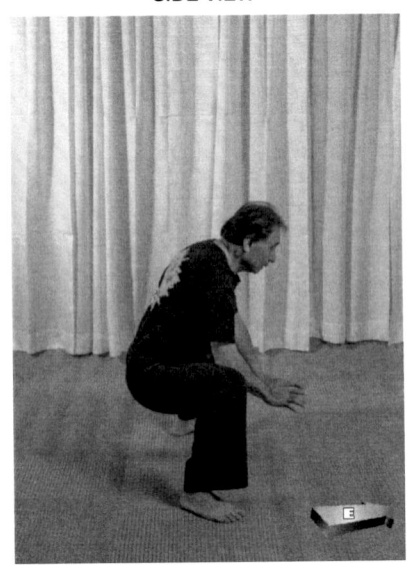

POSTURE 12-*EXHALE*
Both hands press palms down to inside of thigh as you sink weight, bending at knees. Vision follows the hands.

Posture 13

FRONT VIEW

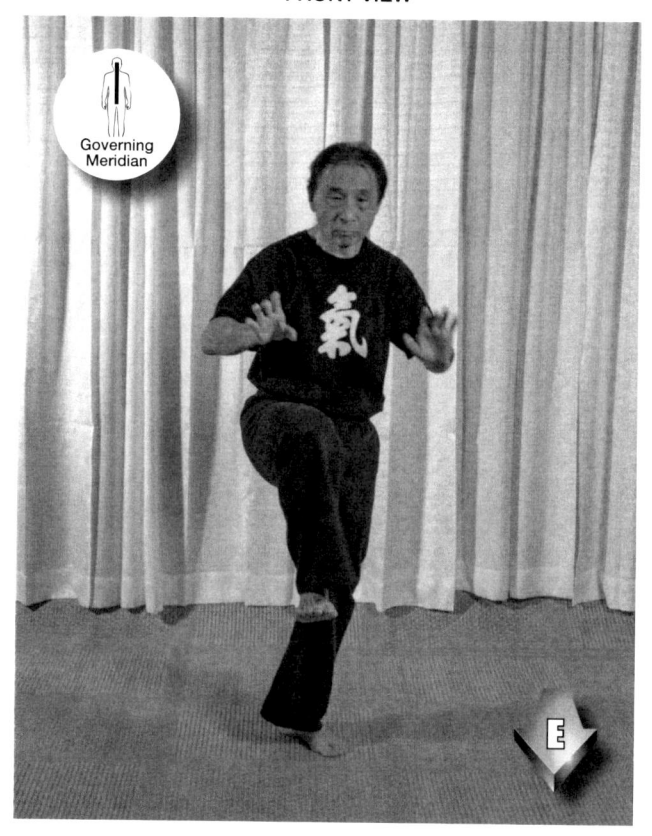

SIDE VIEW

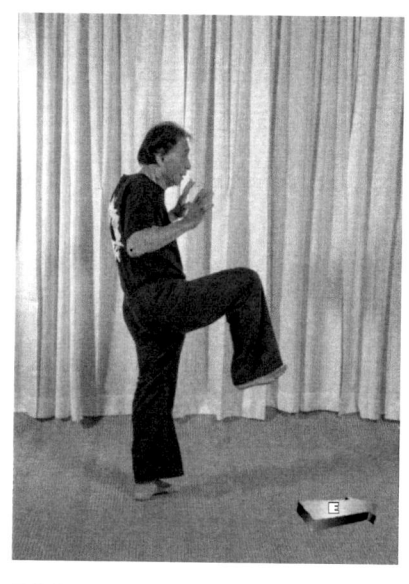

POSTURE 13-*INHALE*
Weight shifts to the left as you bring RF toward left then lift RF up as both hands come to the chest, palms facing forward.

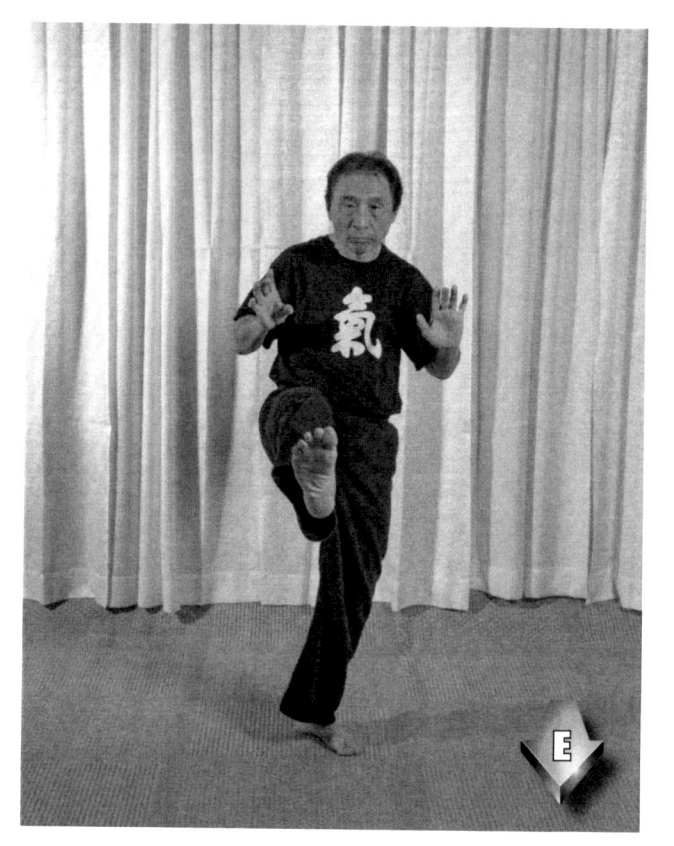

SIDE VIEW

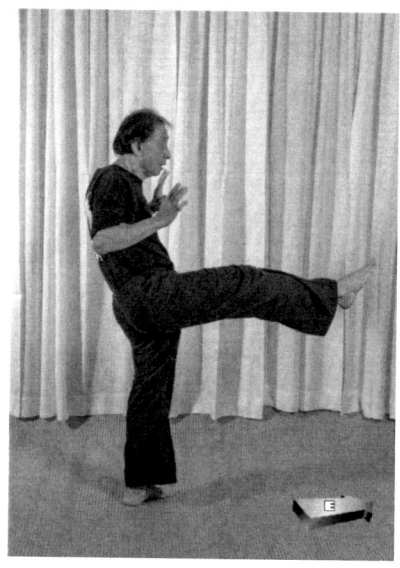

POSTURE 13-*EXHALE*
Extend RF straight to the front, toes pointing forward at end of posture. Hands remain in front of body.

Posture 14

FRONT VIEW

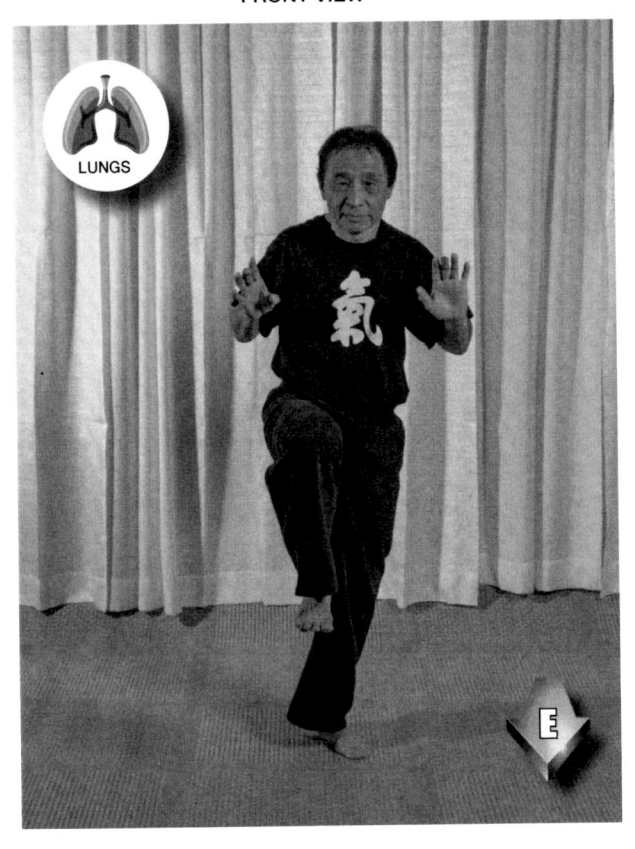

SIDE VIEW

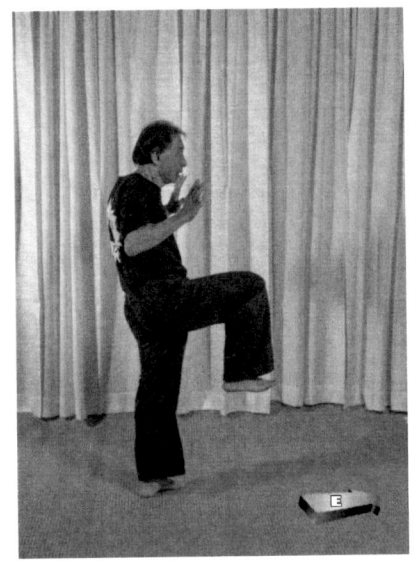

POSTURE 14-_INHALE_
Bring RF back.

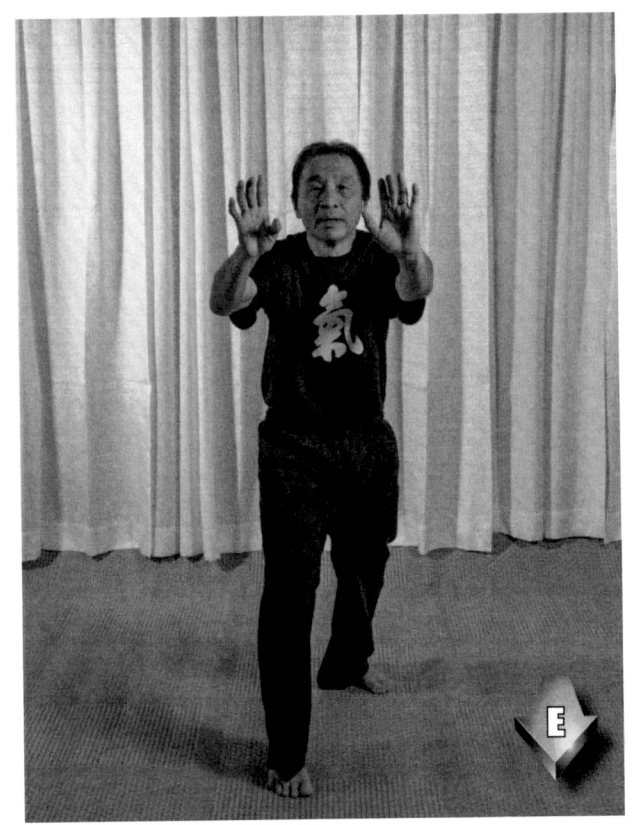

SIDE VIEW

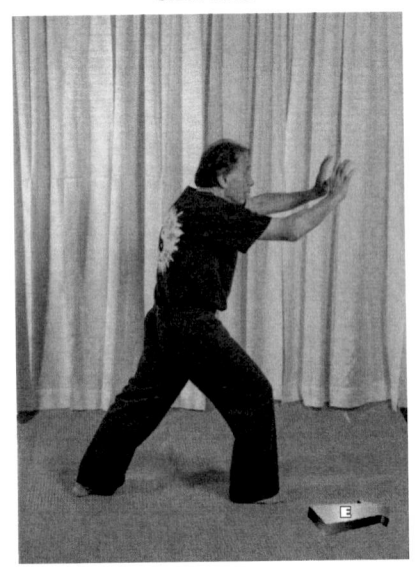

POSTURE 14-_EXHALE_
RF steps forward into BS as both hands press palms forward.

53

Posture 15

FRONT VIEW

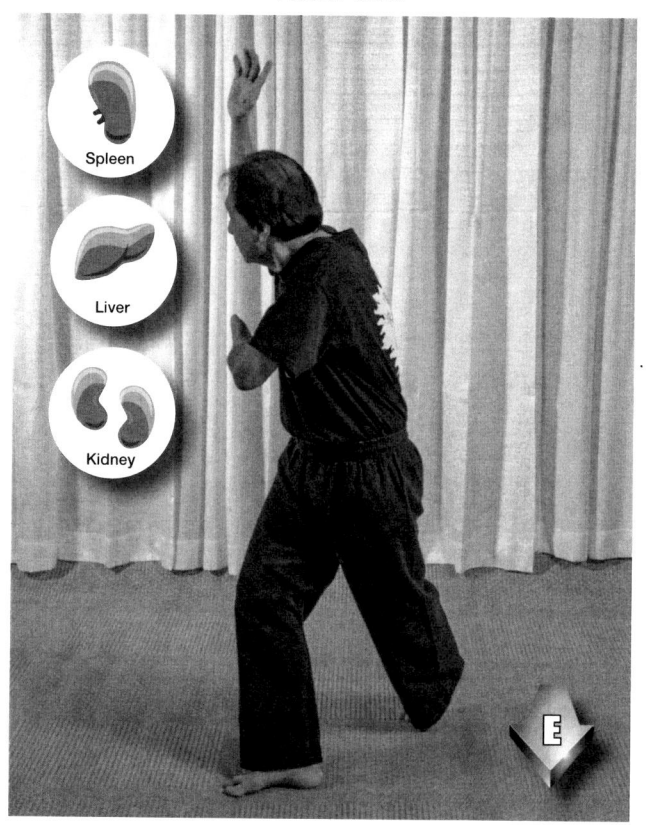

SIDE VIEW

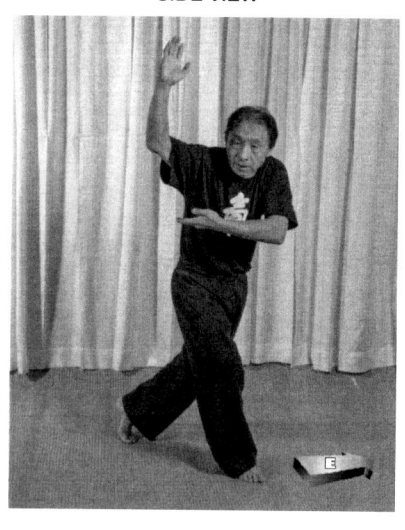

POSTURE 15-*INHALE*
Twist body 180° to the right: RF pivots on heel to the right as the LF pivots on the ball. As you are turning, LH moves under RH, palms facing each other, and both hands follow body around to the right. The RH continues to move toward the rear then moves up with palm facing to the front. LH is at chest, palm up with fingers pointing to right elbow.

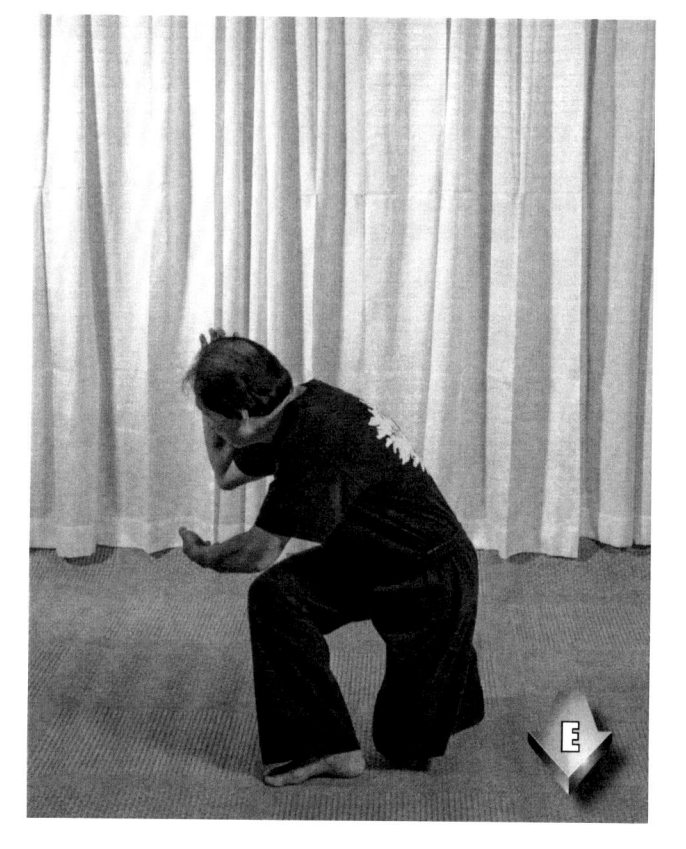

SIDE VIEW

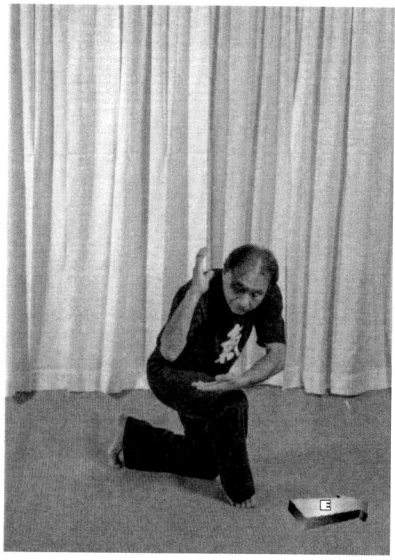

POSTURE 15-*EXHALE*
Sink weight low by bending the knees, keeping arms in same position as you sink. Vision is to the side.

Posture 16

FRONT VIEW

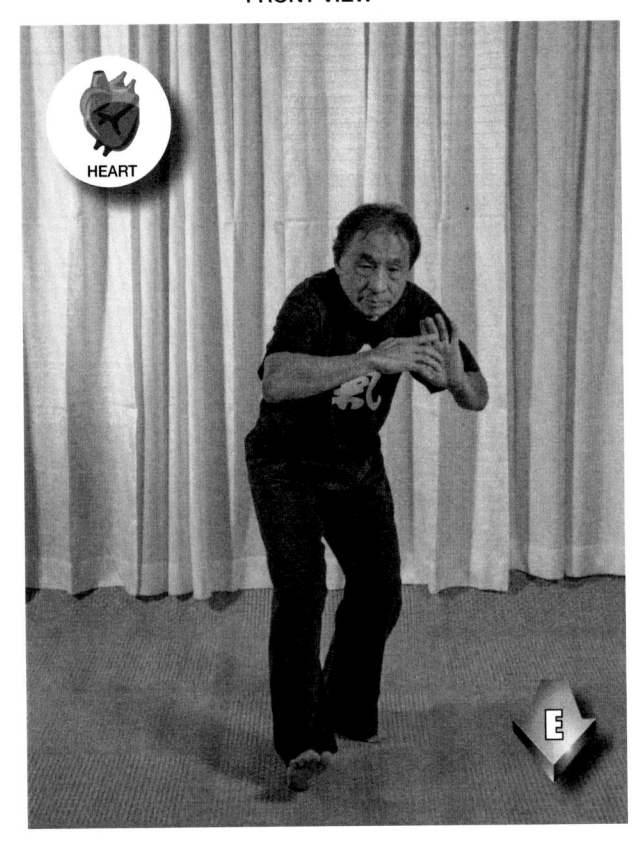

SIDE VIEW

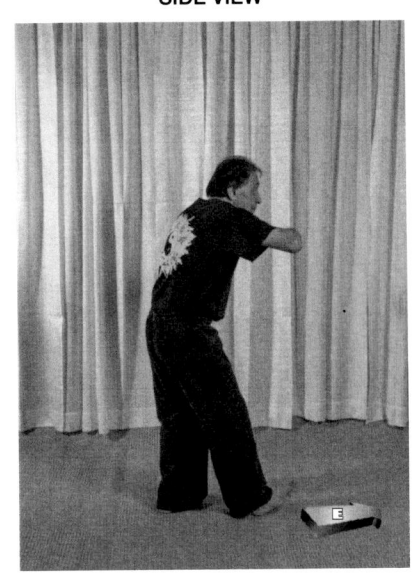

POSTURE 16-*INHALE*
Turn body 180° CCW shifting your weight to the LF as the RF comes back to heel and hands sweep around and come back to chest with RH in front, fingers pointing to the left and LH behind with fingers pointing up.

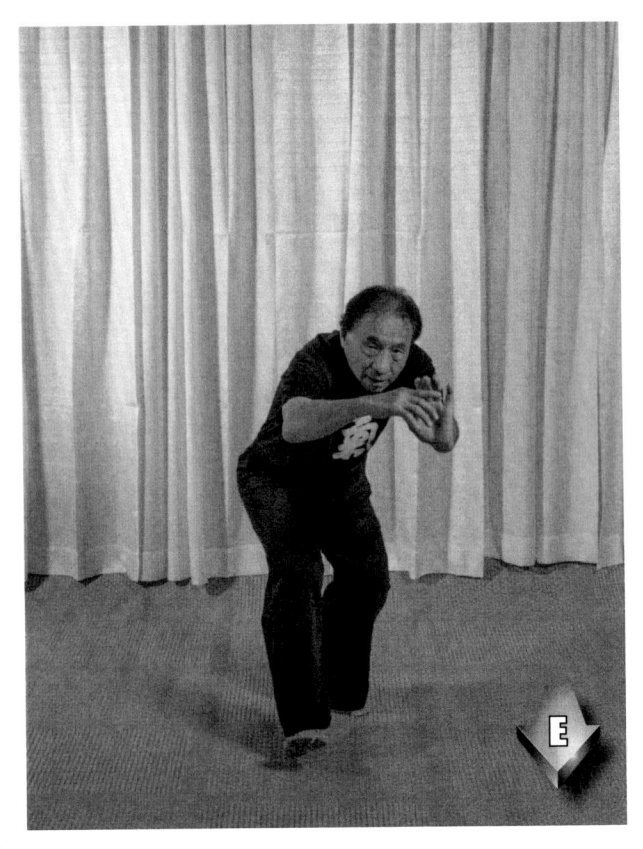

SIDE VIEW

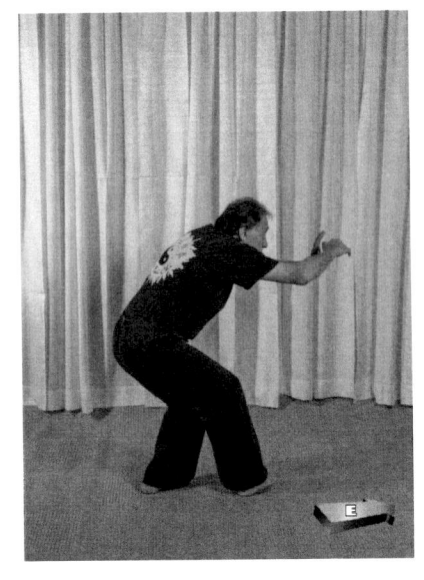

POSTURE 16-*EXHALE*
Sink down in heel stance as hands extend forward. Keep elbows up.

Posture 17

FRONT VIEW

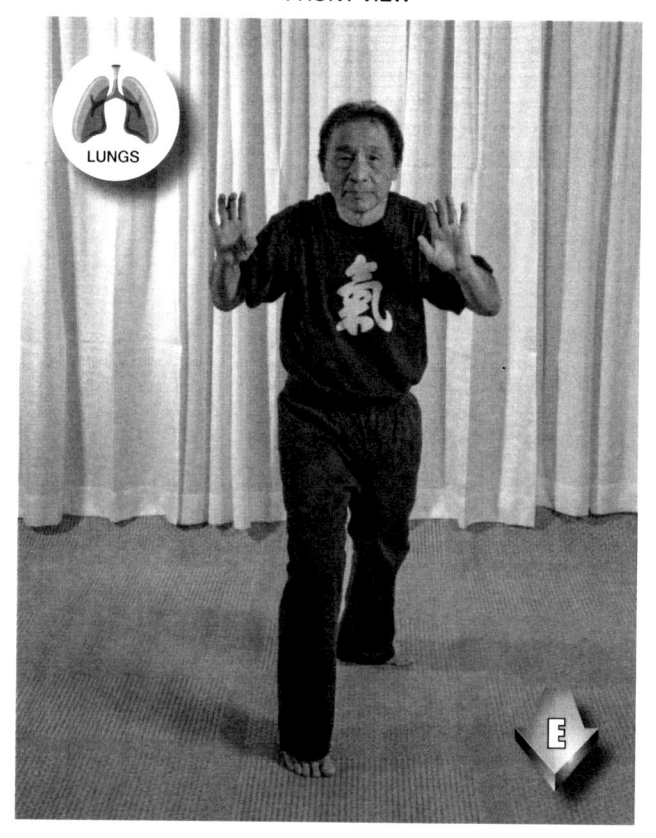

SIDE VIEW

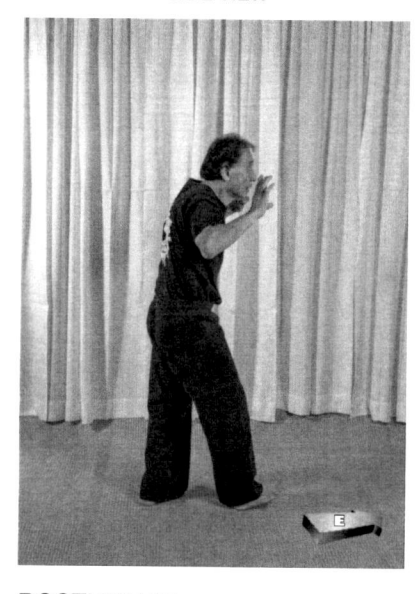

POSTURE 17-*INHALE*
Pull hands back to shoulder height, palms facing forward.

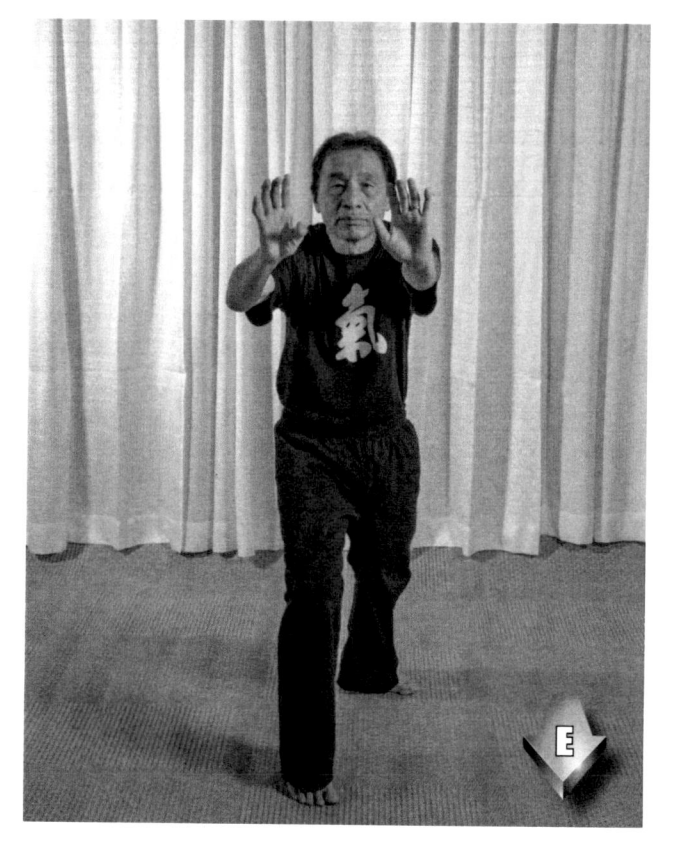

SIDE VIEW

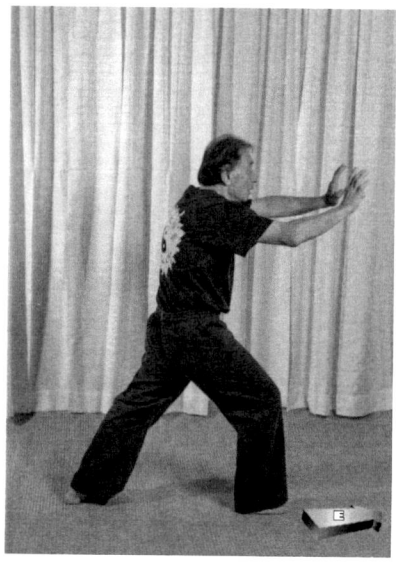

POSTURE 17-*EXHALE*
RF steps forward into BS as both hands extend to the front, palms facing forward.

Posture 18

FRONT VIEW

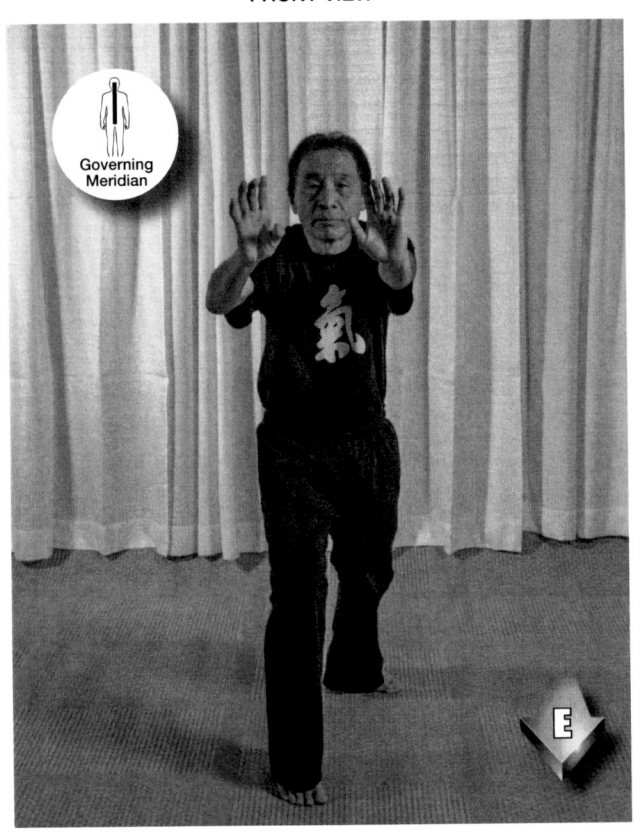

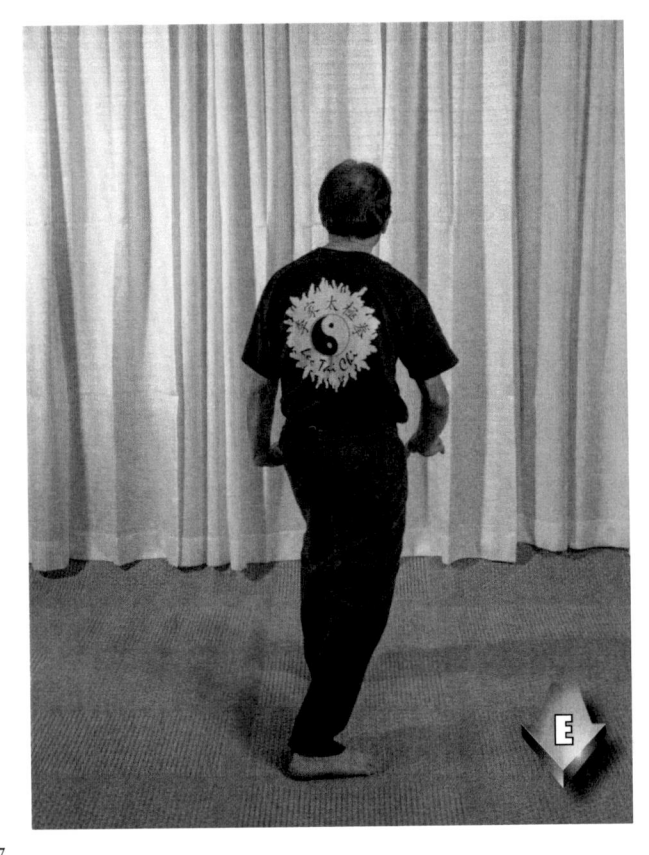

POSTURE 18-*INHALE*

Turn body 180° CCW with hands extended out to the front, palms down. Weight shifts from RF forward to LF forward as you turn. Finish by making CW half circle with both arms, palms forward, ending with both hands out in front of body, above head, palms down.

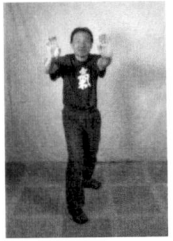

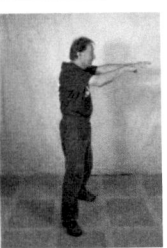

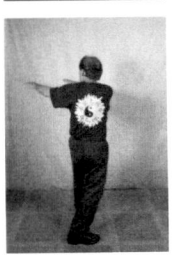

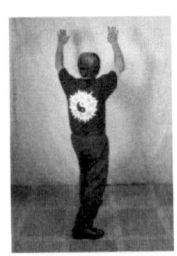

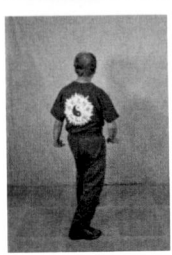

POSTURE 18-*EXHALE*

Hands move down to sides of body and slightly outward to each side. Palms face downward.

Posture 19

FRONT VIEW

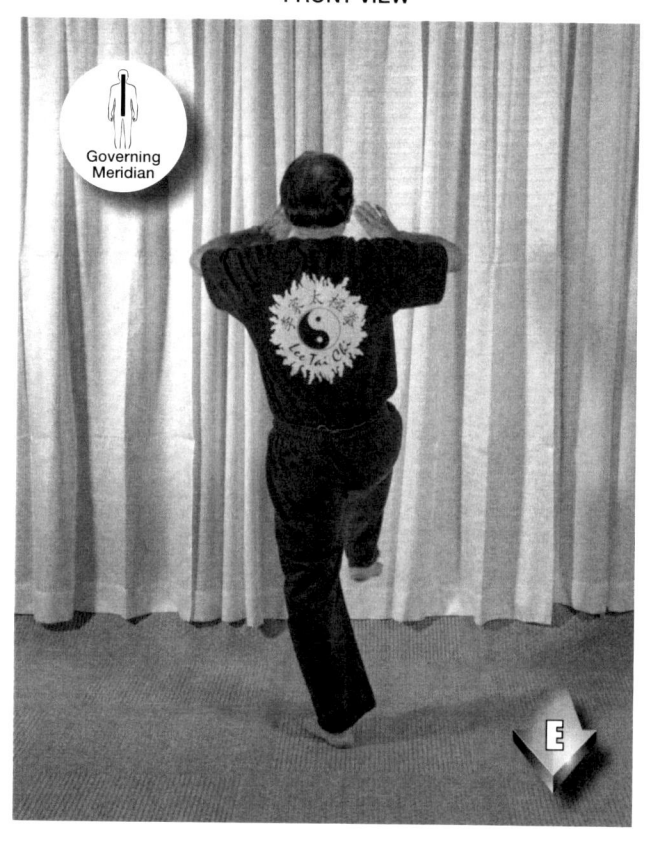

POSTURE 19-*INHALE*

RF moves forward and raises up as the hands move up together, palms forward, forming a triangular shape above head height. Arms do not cross, vision follows hands looking through triangular opening.

Sequential reverse view

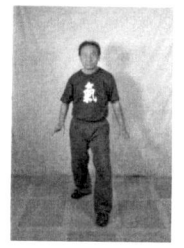

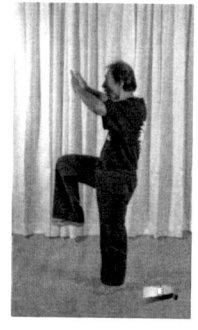

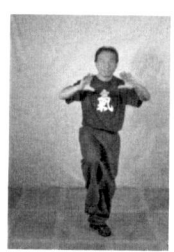

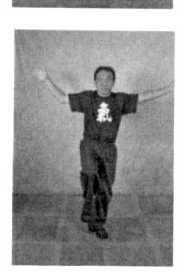

SIDE VIEW

SIDE VIEW

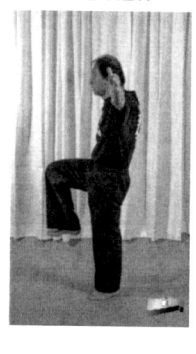

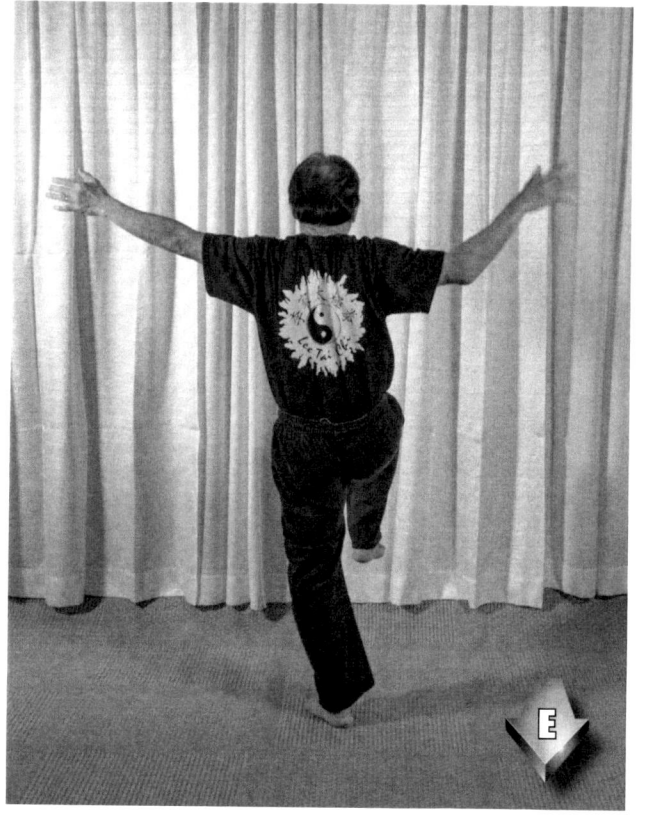

POSTURE 19-*EXHALE*

Hands continue to circle to the outside and down to shoulder level, palms facing forward.

Posture 20

FRONT VIEW

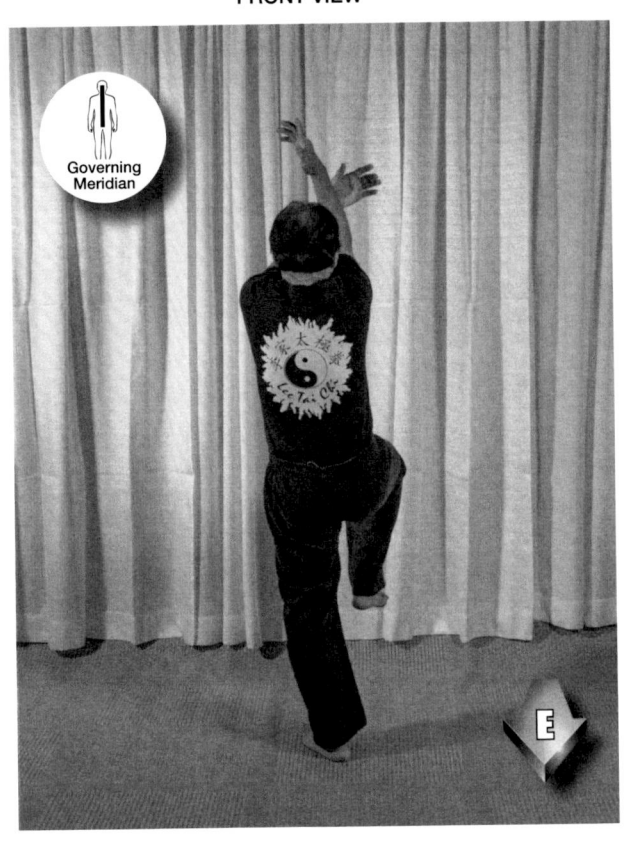

POSTURE 20-*INHALE*
Hands circle back up to over the head, palms turning to the rear, then cross arms with RH behind the left.

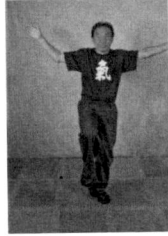

Sequential reverse view

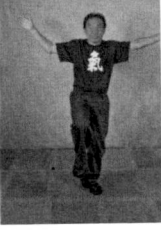

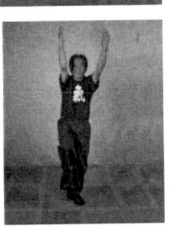

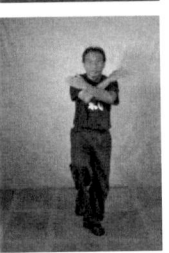

SIDE VIEW

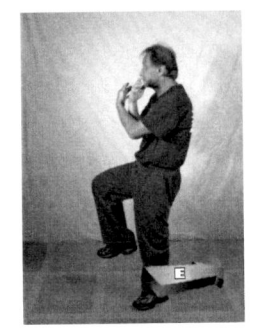

SIDE VIEW

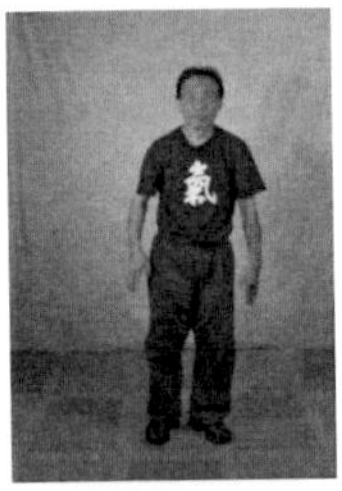

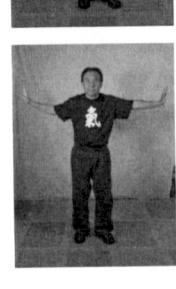

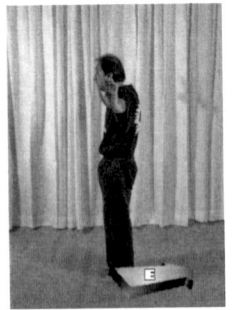

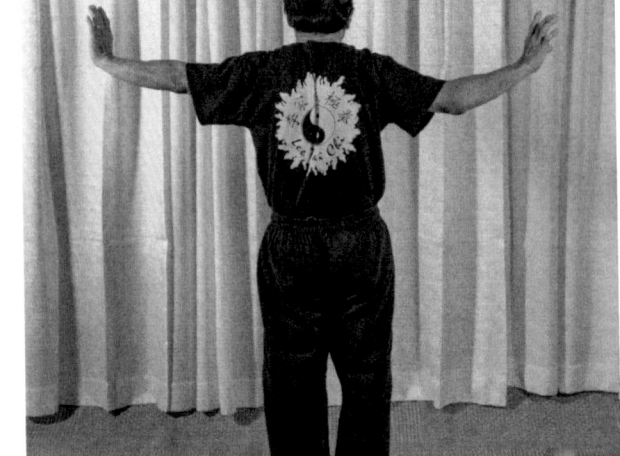

POSTURE 20-*EXHALE*
RF down as hands continue move downward in front of body, turning palms down so right arm is on top of left in front of body. Continue to move arms down and then up and out to the side to shoulder level, wrists bent and fingertips up.

Governing Meridian

Posture 21

FRONT VIEW

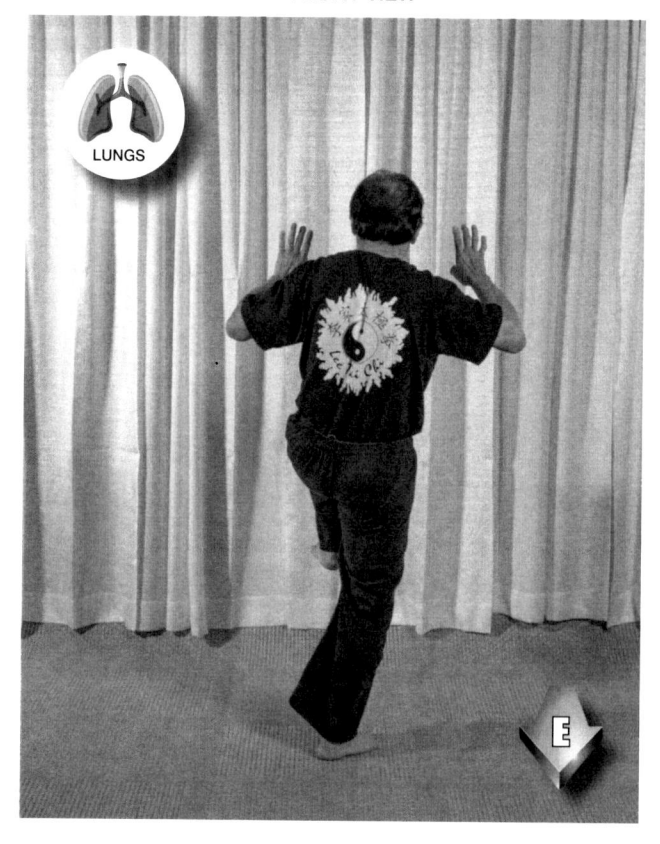

SIDE VIEW

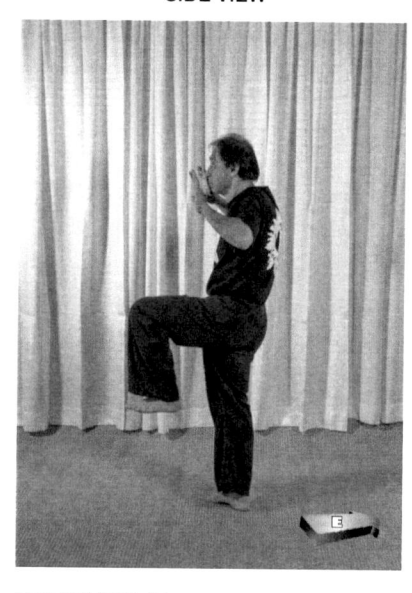

POSTURE 21-*INHALE*
Shift weight to right, then hands come in towards body at shoulder level, palms forward as you raise LF.

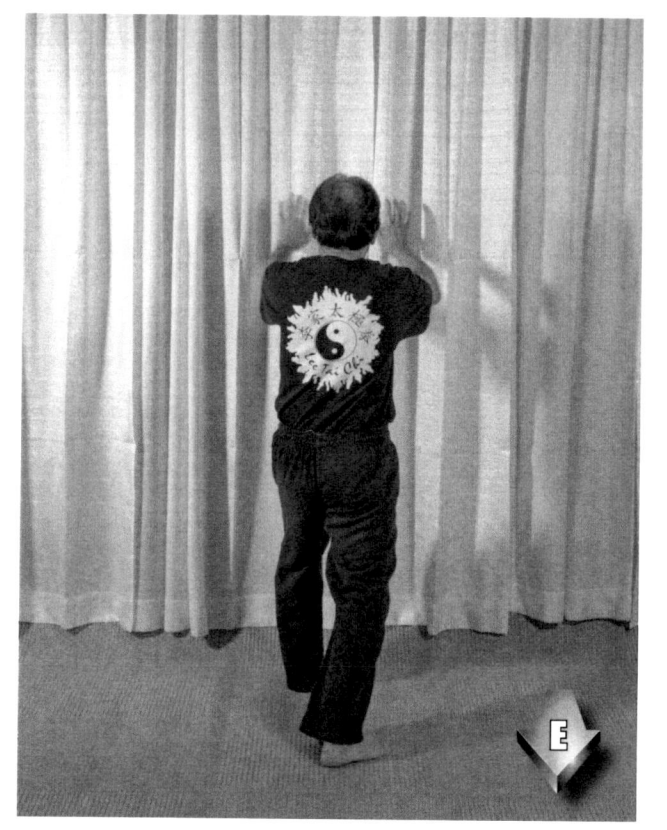

SIDE VIEW

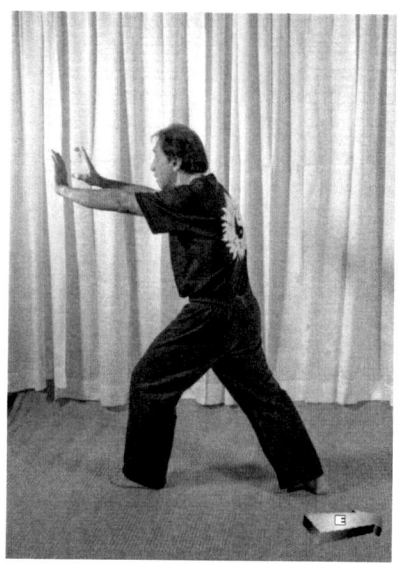

POSTURE 21-*EXHALE*
LF steps forward into BS as hands extend to the front with the palms facing forward.

60

Posture 22

FRONT VIEW

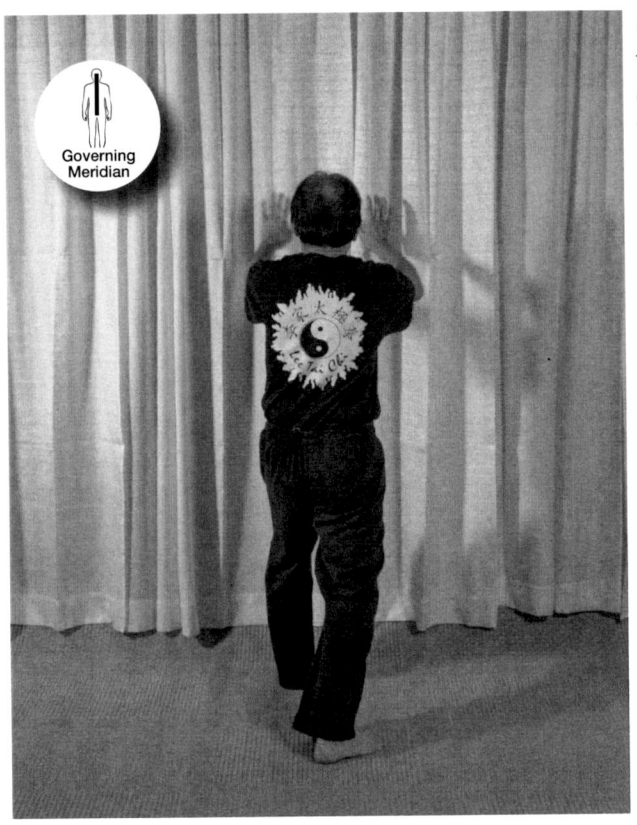

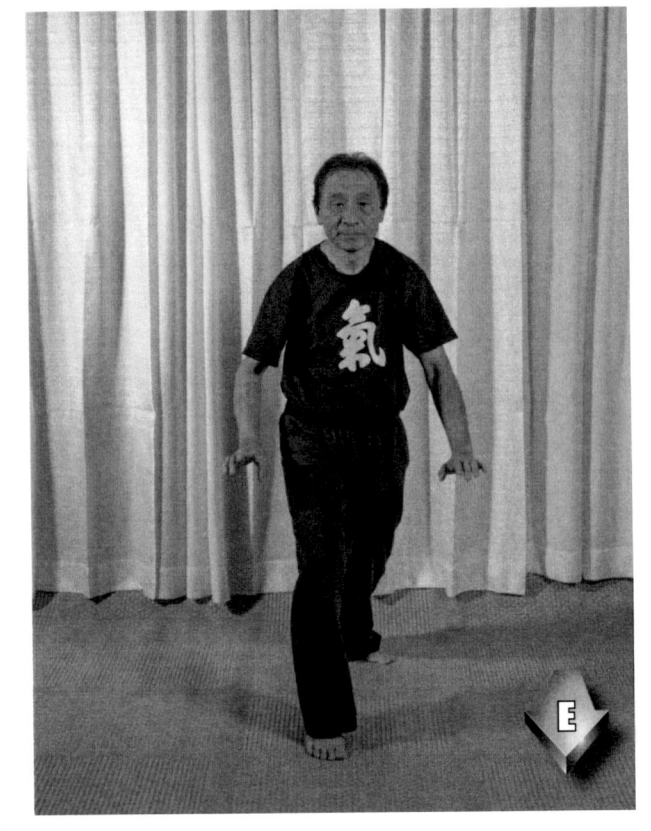

POSTURE 22-*INHALE*
Turn body 180° CW with hands extended out to the front, palms down. (Weight shifts from LF forward to RF forward as you turn) Finish by making CCW half circle with both arms, palms forward, ending with both hands out in front of body, above head.

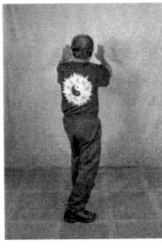

Sequential view

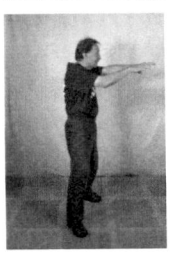

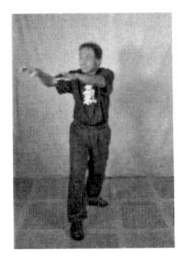

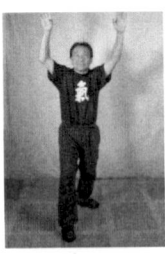

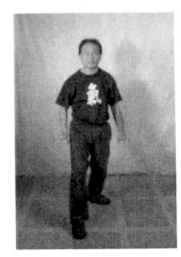

POSTURE 22-*EXHALE*
Hands move down to sides of body and slightly outward to each side. Palms face down.

Posture 23

FRONT VIEW

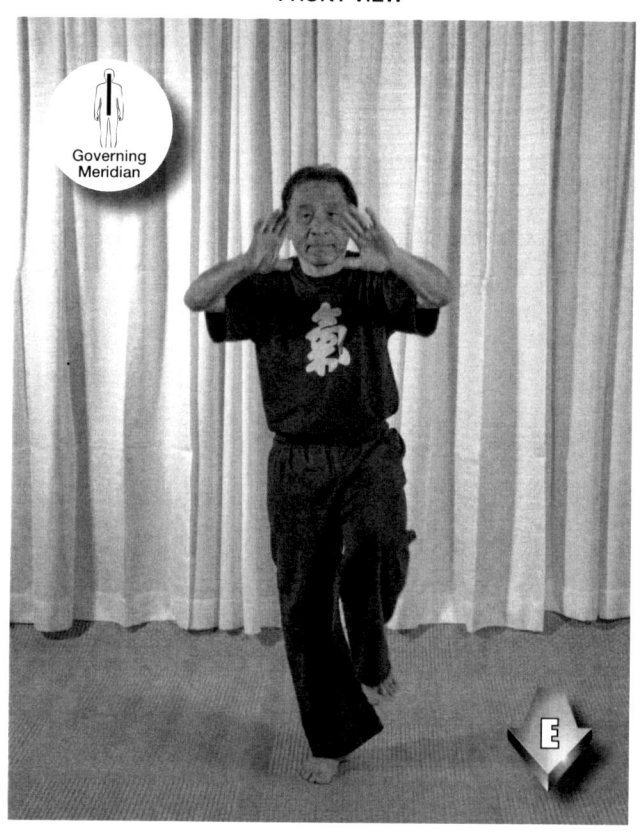

POSTURE 23-*INHALE*

LF moves forward and raises up as the hands move up together, palms forward, forming a triangular shape above head height. Arms do not cross, vision follows hands looking through triangular opening.

Sequential view   SIDE VIEW

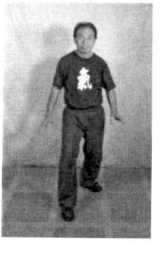

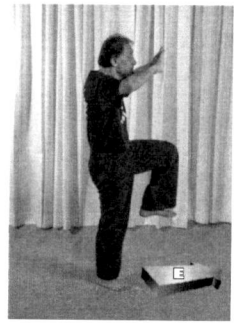

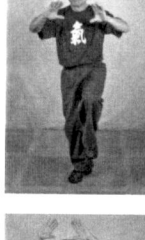

SIDE VIEW

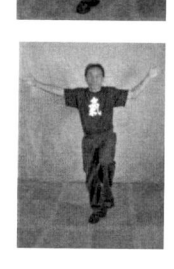

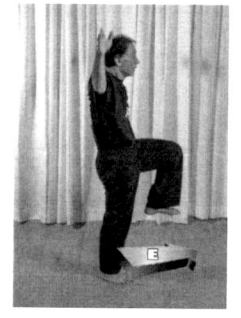

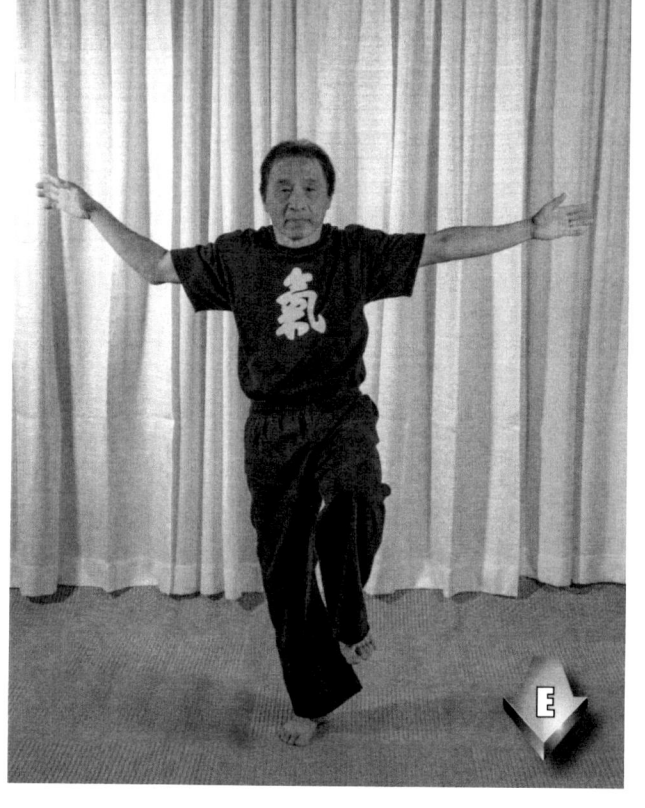

POSTURE 23-*EXHALE*

Hands continue to circle to the outside and down to shoulder level, palms facing forward.

Posture 24

FRONT VIEW

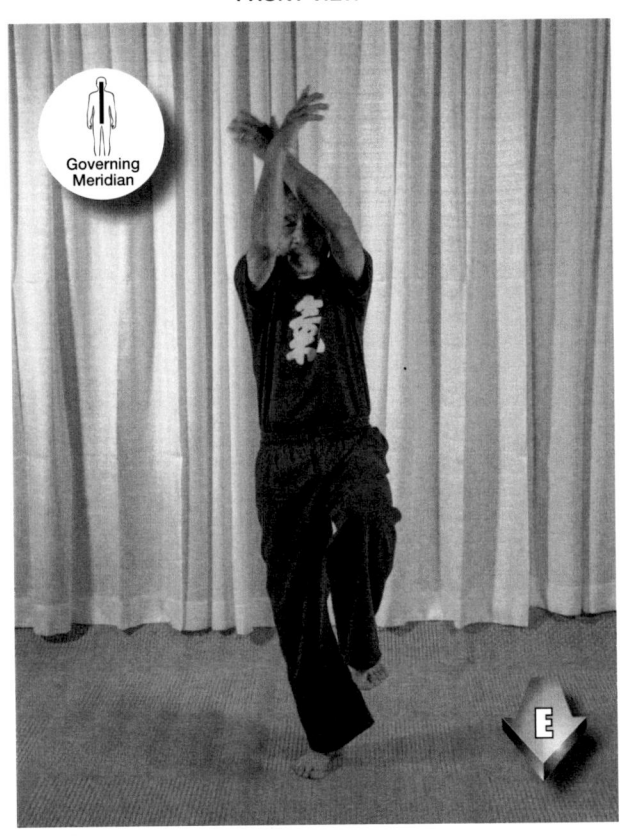

POSTURE 24-*INHALE*
Hands circle back up to over the head, palms turning to the rear, then cross arms with LH behind the RH.

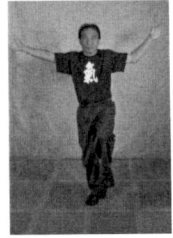

Sequential view

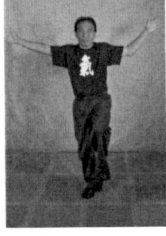

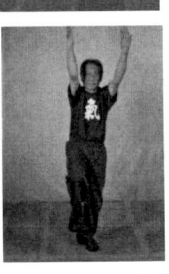

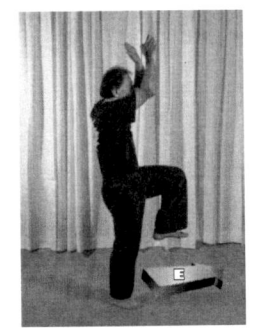

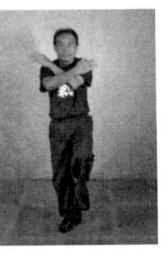

SIDE VIEW

SIDE VIEW

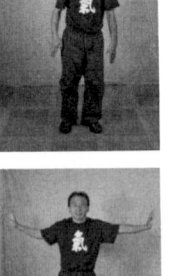

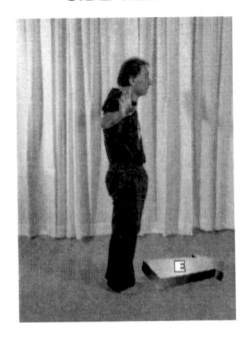

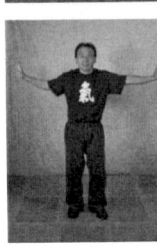

POSTURE 24-*EXHALE*
LF down as hands continue move downward in front of body, turning palms down so left arm is on top of right in front of body. Continue to move arms down and then up and out to the side to shoulder level, wrists bent and fingertips up.

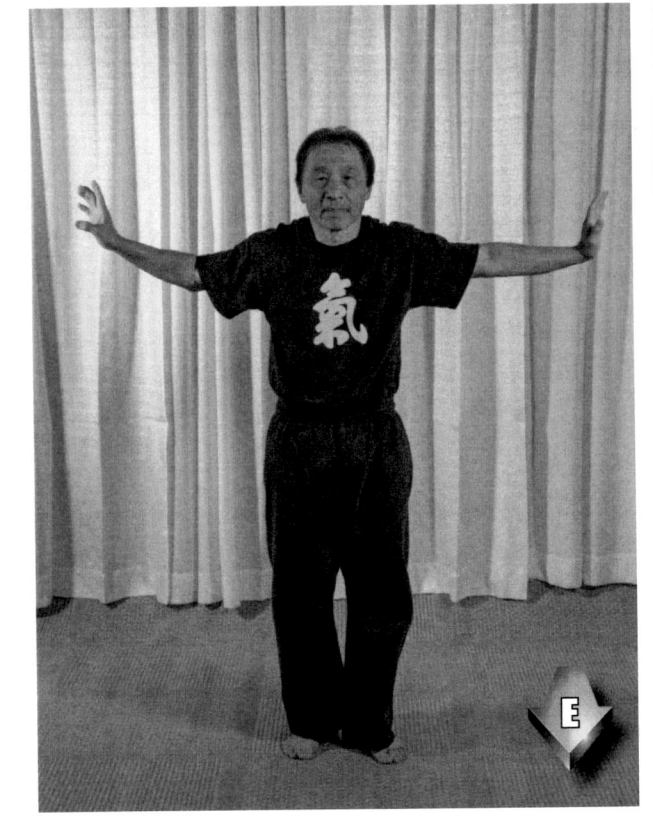

Posture 25

FRONT VIEW

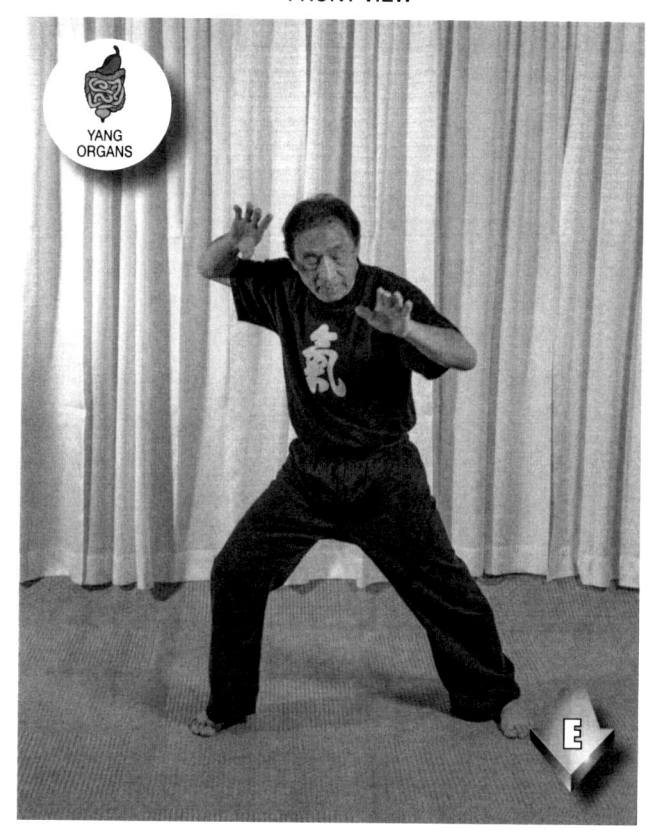

SIDE VIEW

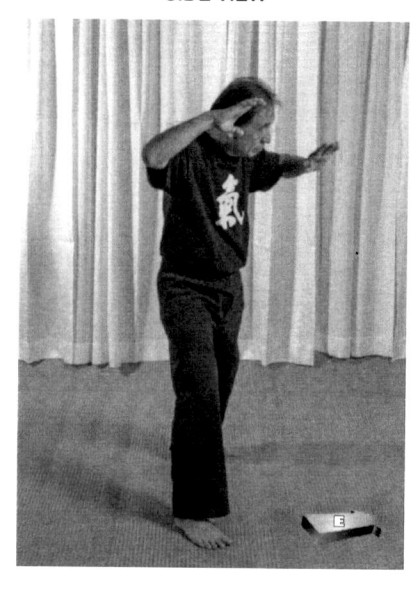

POSTURE 25-*INHALE*
LH moves into left temple as LF lifts and steps out to the left side. RH comes in toward right temple

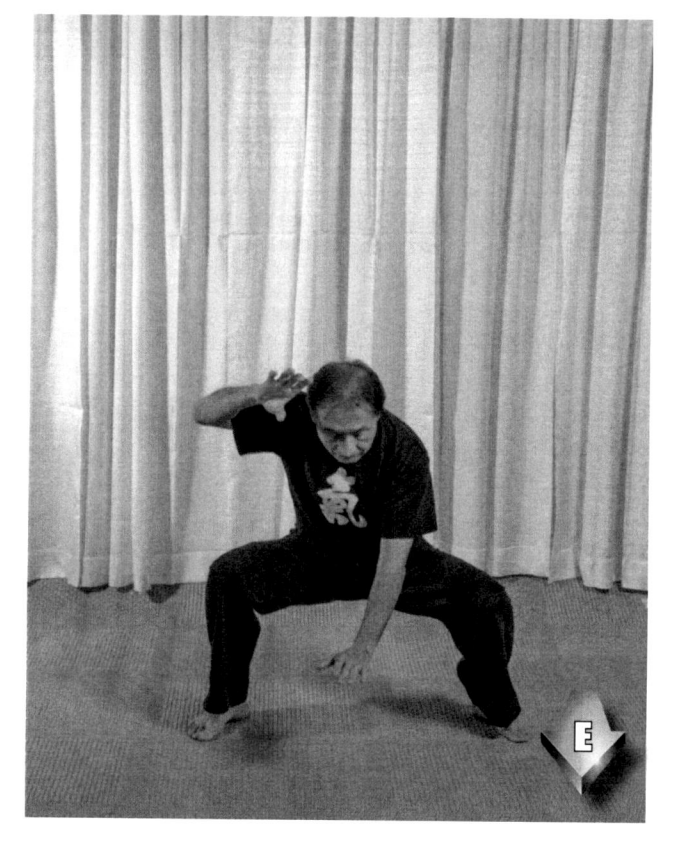

SIDE VIEW

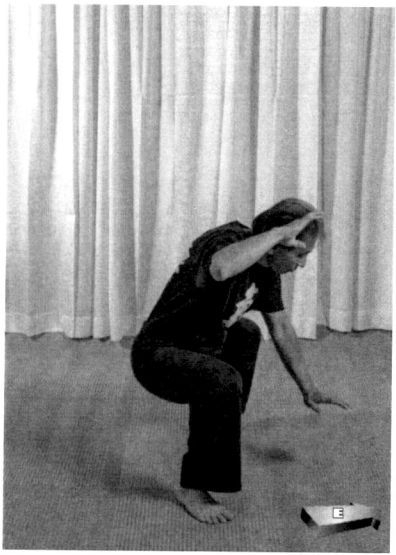

POSTURE 25-*EXHALE*
Left palm presses down to floor between legs. RH remains at right temple. Vision follows left hand.

Posture 26

FRONT VIEW

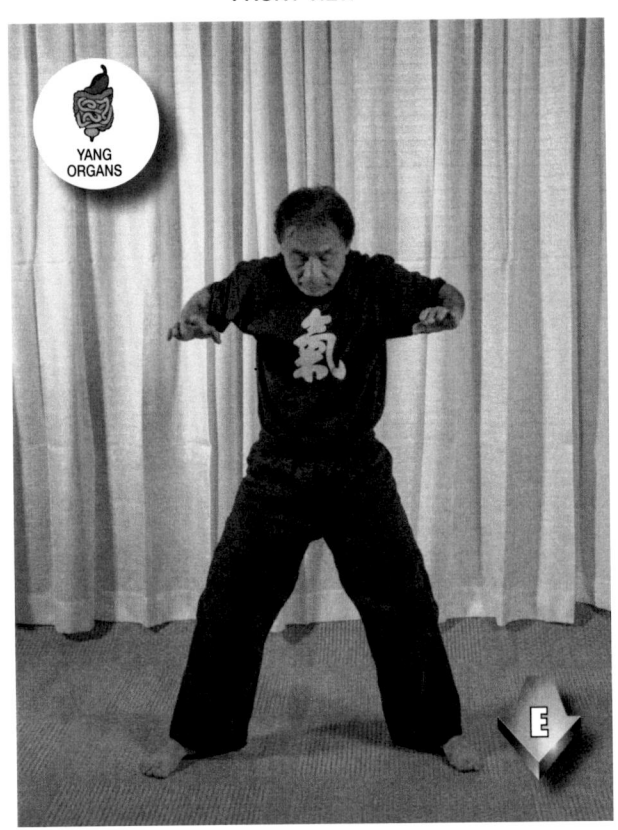

SIDE VIEW

YANG ORGANS

Circle hands sequence

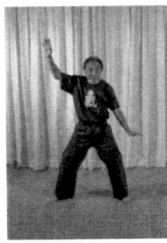

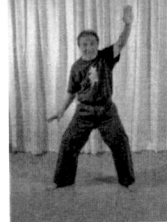

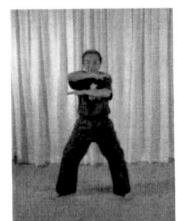

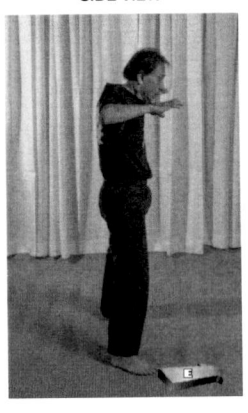

POSTURE
26-*INHALE*

RH extends out to the right as both hands circle in CW direction and cross in front of body, LH crosses in front. (Body turns facing the front into HS as you circle hands) then both hands pull rearward, palms down, as you expand the chest.

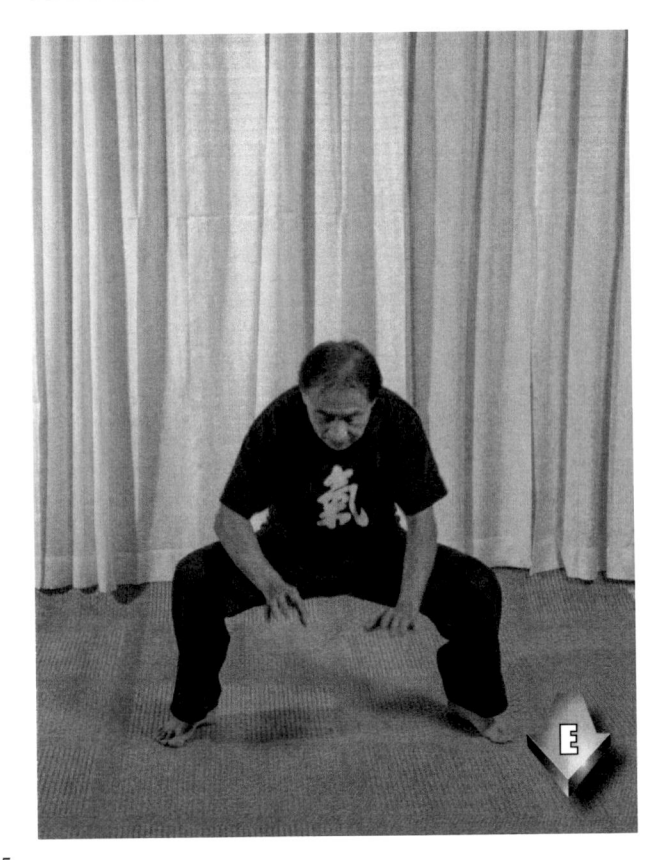

SIDE VIEW

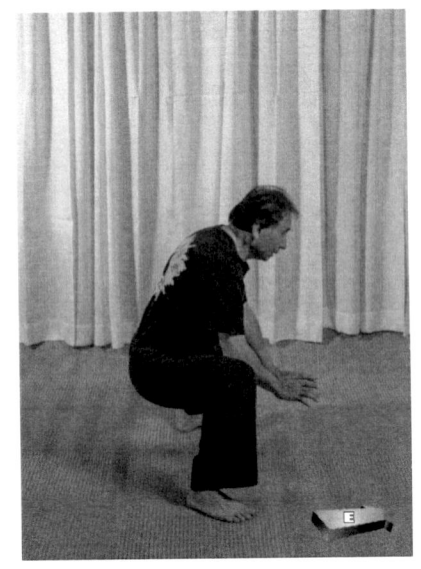

POSTURE 26-*EXHALE*

Both hands press palm down to inside of thigh as you sink weight, bending at knees. Vision follows the hands.

Posture 27

FRONT VIEW

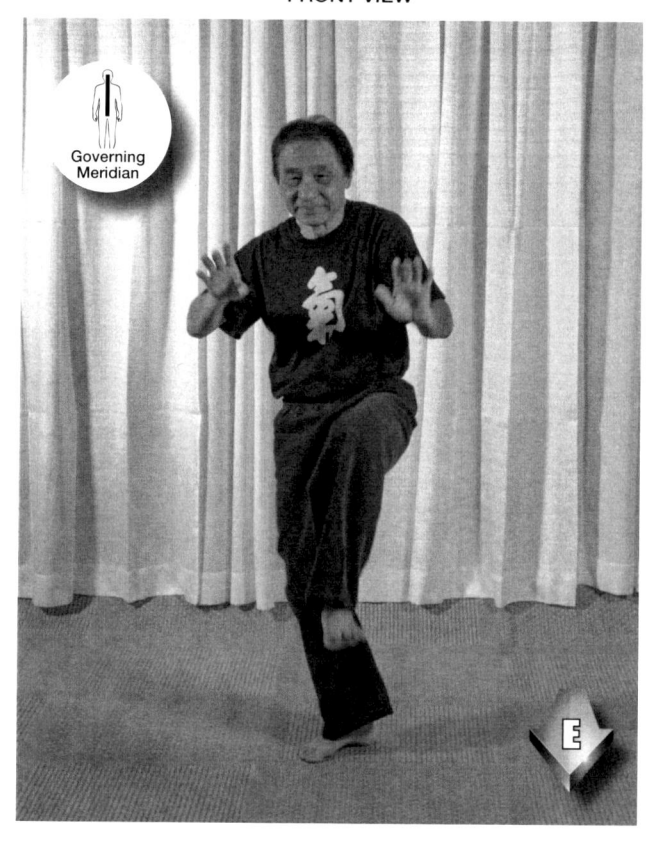

Governing Meridian

SIDE VIEW

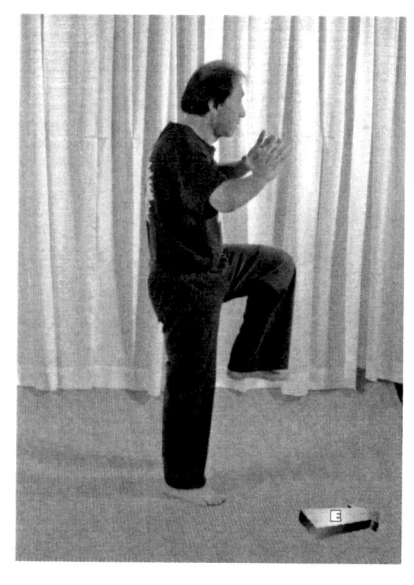

POSTURE 27-*INHALE*
Weight shifts to the right as you bring LF toward right then lift LF up as both hands come to the chest, palms facing forward.

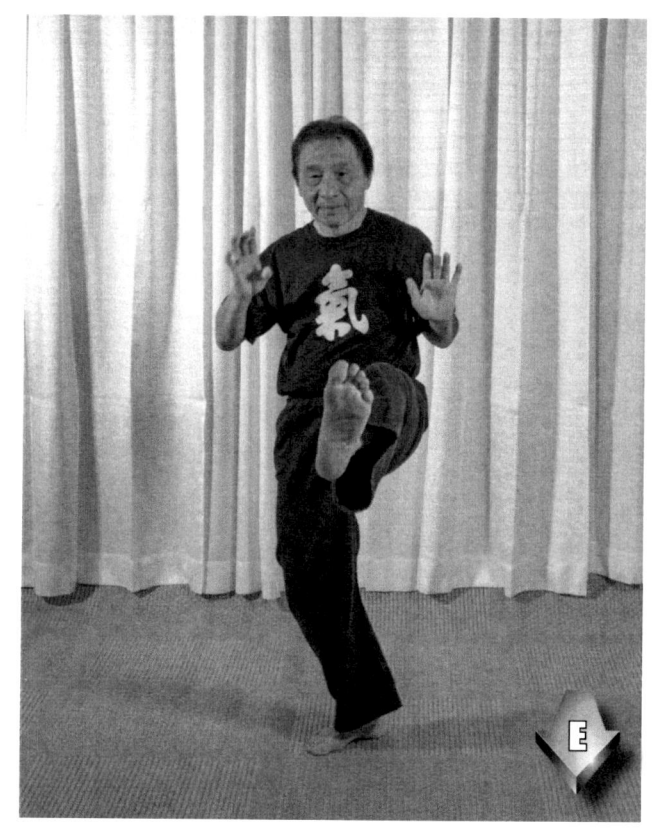

SIDE VIEW

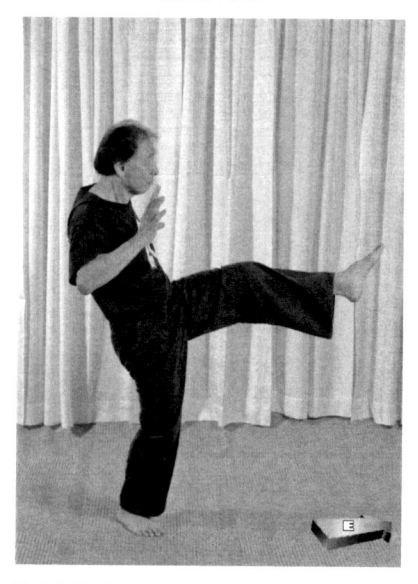

POSTURE 27-*EXHALE*
Extend LF straight to the front, toes pointing forward at end of posture. Hands remain in front of body.

Posture 28

FRONT VIEW

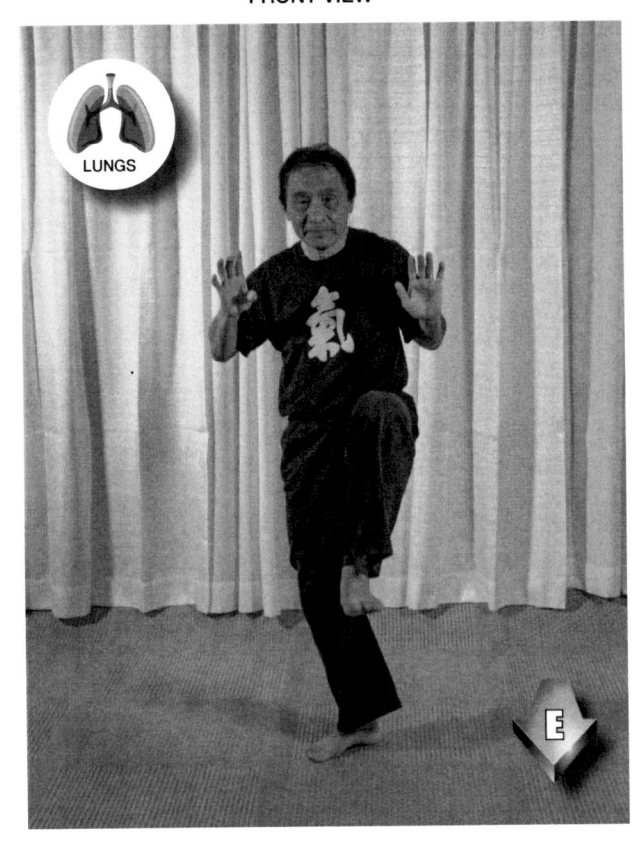

SIDE VIEW

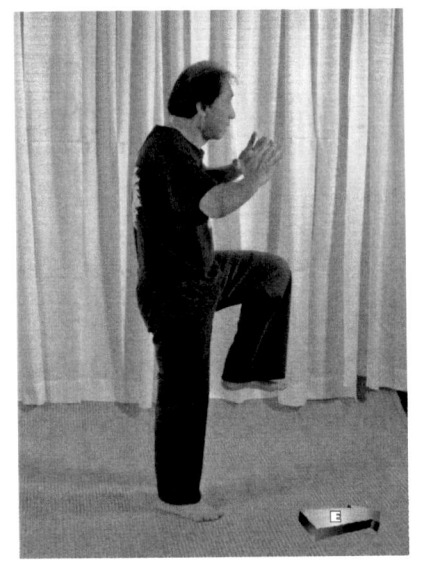

POSTURE 28-*INHALE*
Bring LF back.

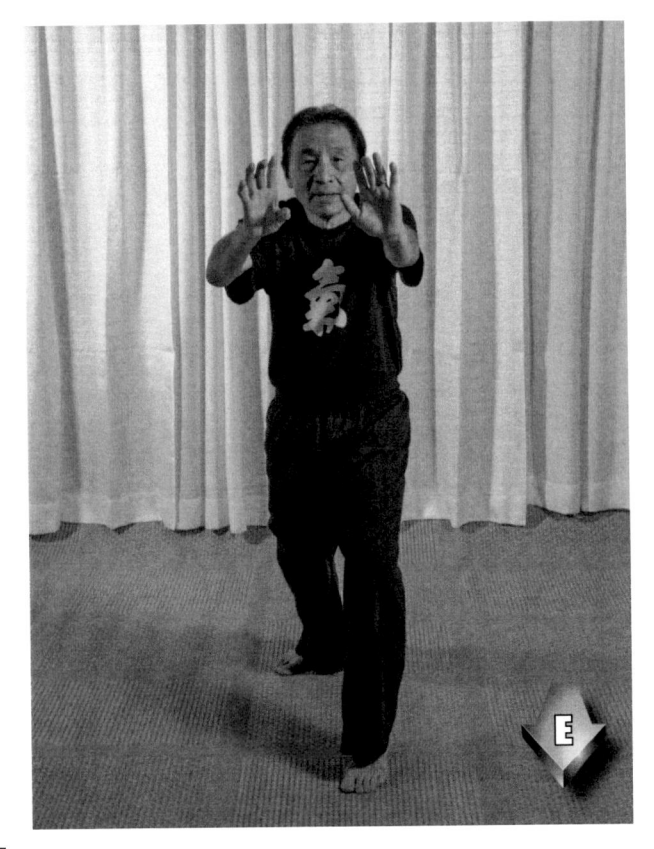

SIDE VIEW

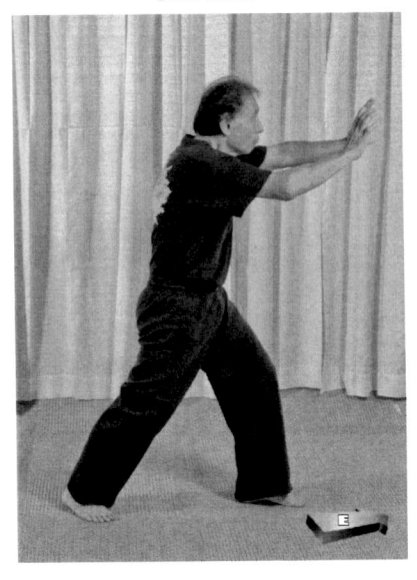

POSTURE 28-*EXHALE*
LF steps forward into BS as both hands extend to the front, palms forward.

Posture 29

FRONT VIEW

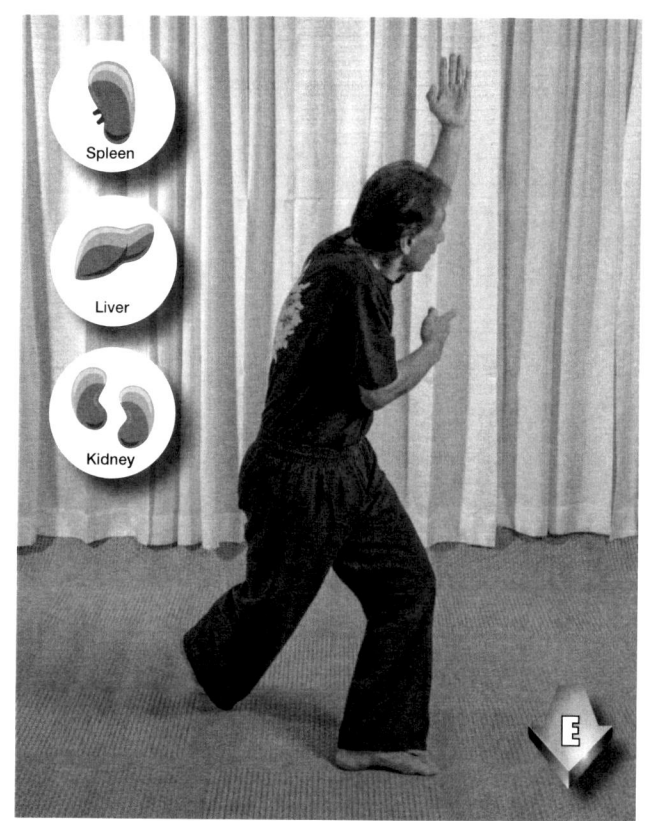

SIDE VIEW

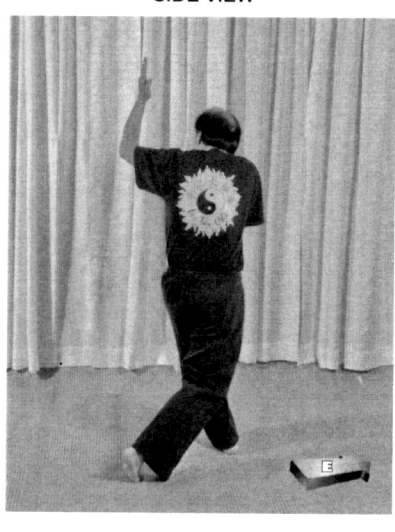

POSTURE 29-*INHALE*

Twist body 180° to the left: LF pivots on heel to the right as the RF pivots on the ball. As you are turning, RH moves under LH, palms facing each other, and both hands follow body around to the left. The LH continues to move toward the rear then moves up with palm facing to the front. RH is at chest, palm up with fingers pointing to left elbow.

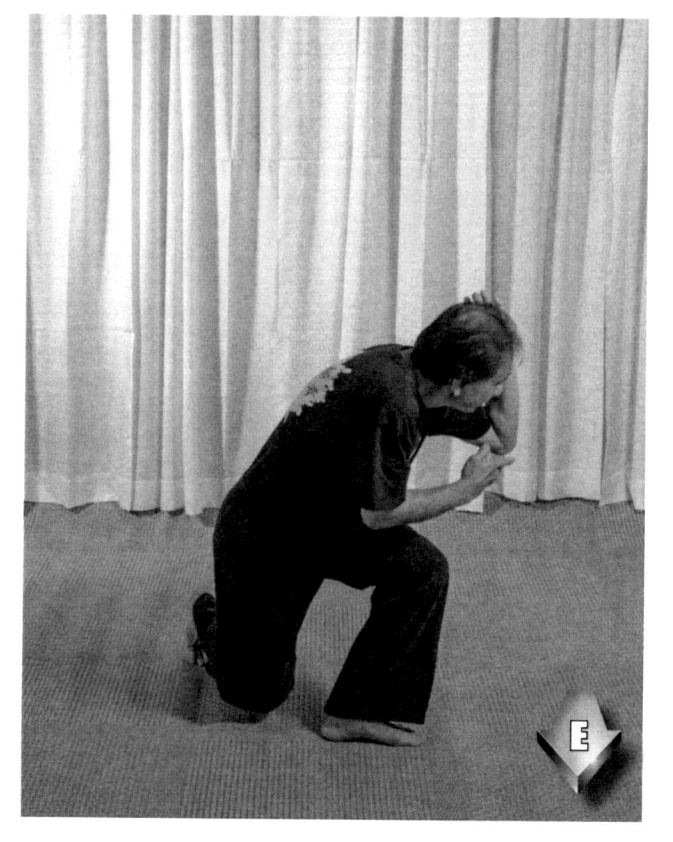

SIDE VIEW

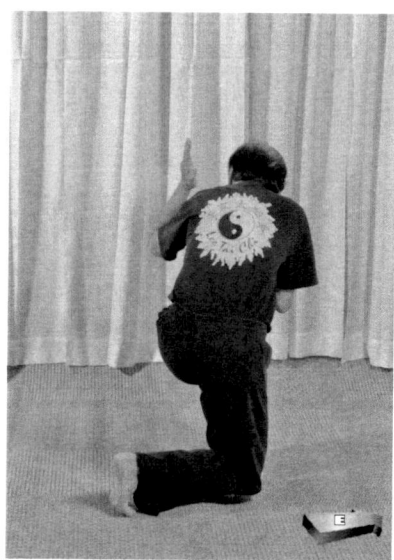

POSTURE 29-*EXHALE*

Sink weight low by bending the knees, keeping arms in same position as you sink. Vision is to the side.

Posture 30

FRONT VIEW

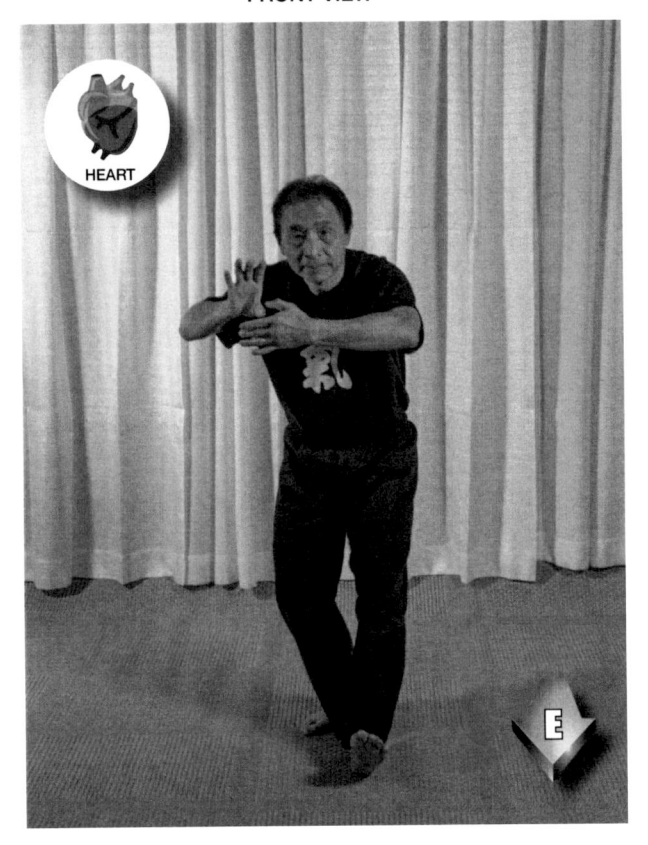

SIDE VIEW

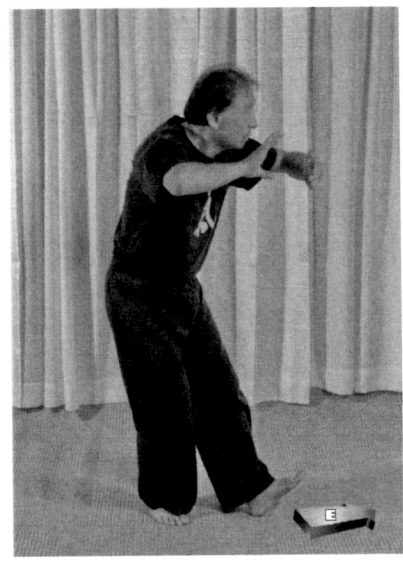

POSTURE 30-*INHALE*
Turn body 180° CW shifting your weight to the RF as the LF comes back to heel and hands sweep around and come back to chest with LH in front, fingers pointing to the left and RH behind with fingers pointing up.

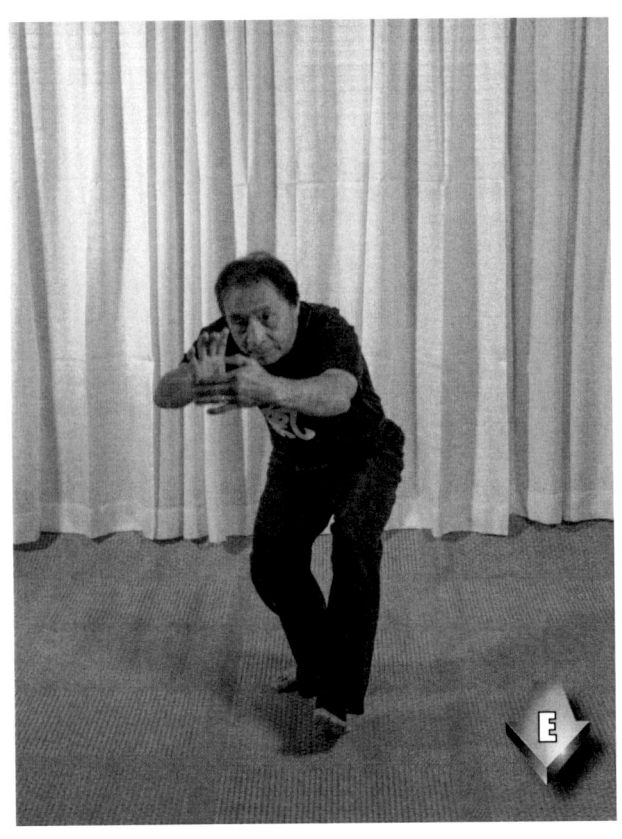

SIDE VIEW

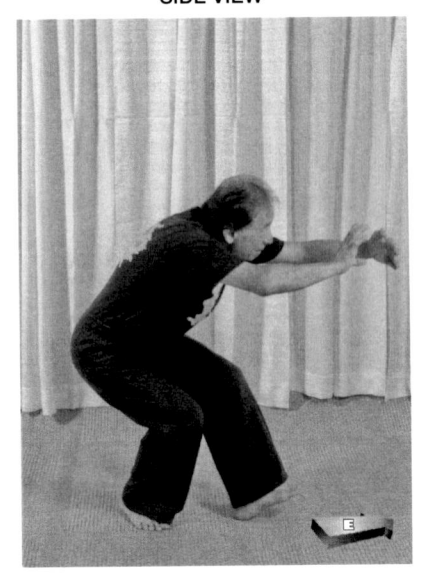

POSTURE 30-*EXHALE*
Sink down in heel stance as hands extend forward. Keep elbows up.

Posture 31

FRONT VIEW

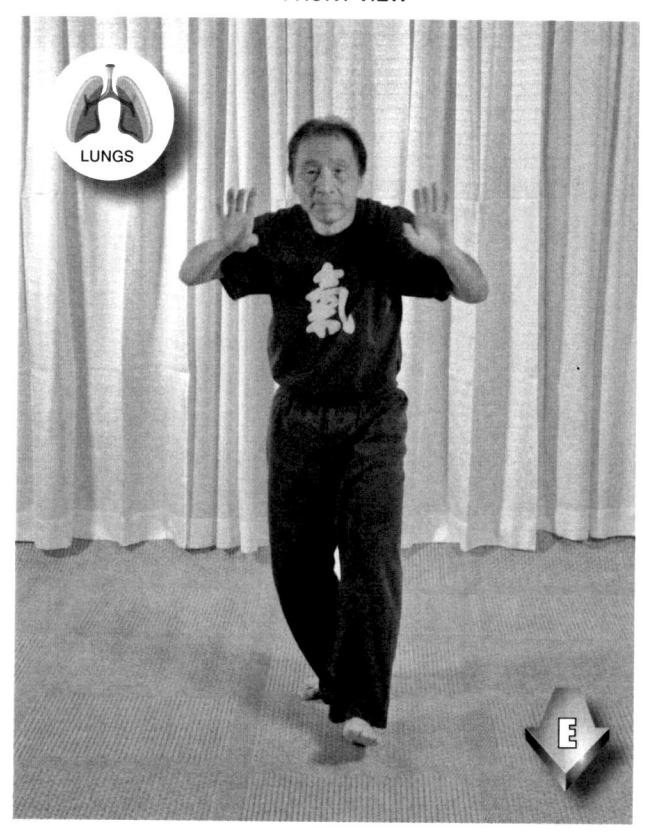

SIDE VIEW

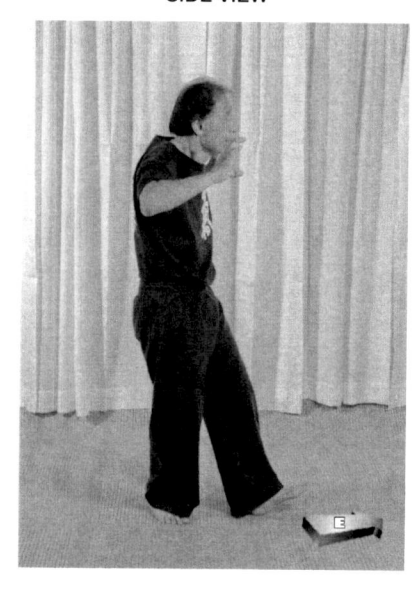

POSTURE 31 -*INHALE*
Pull hands back to shoulder height, palms facing forward.

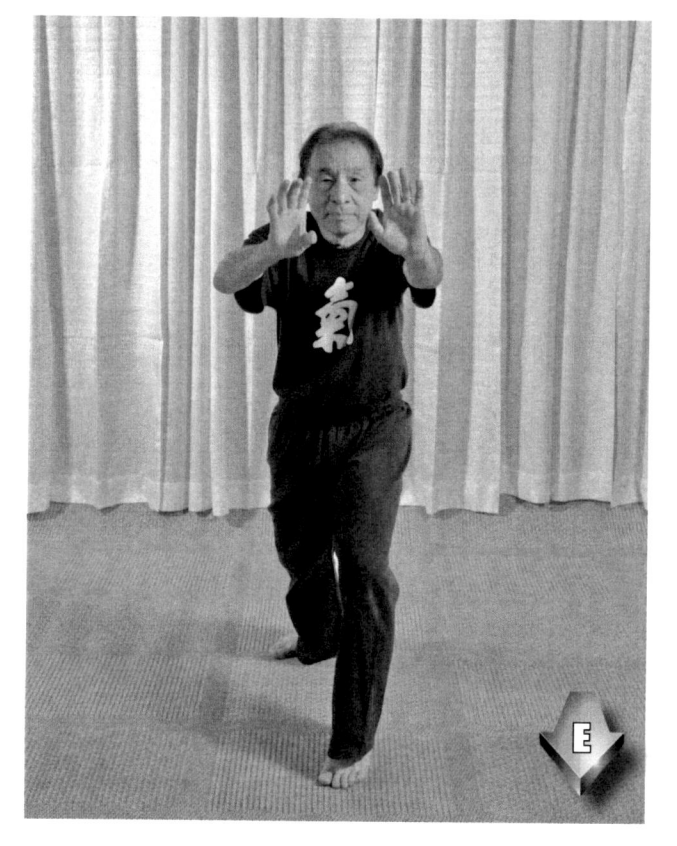

SIDE VIEW

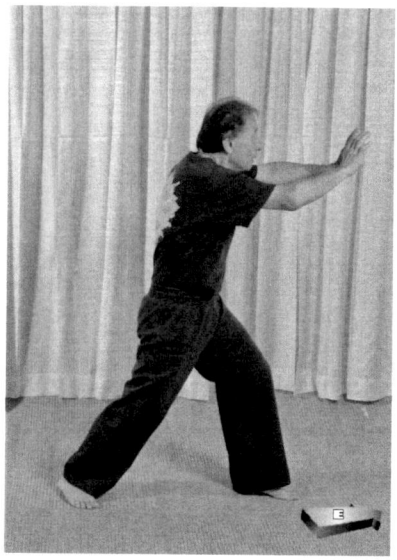

POSTURE 31 -*EXHALE*
LF steps forward into BS as both hands extend to the front, palms facing forward.

Posture 32

FRONT VIEW

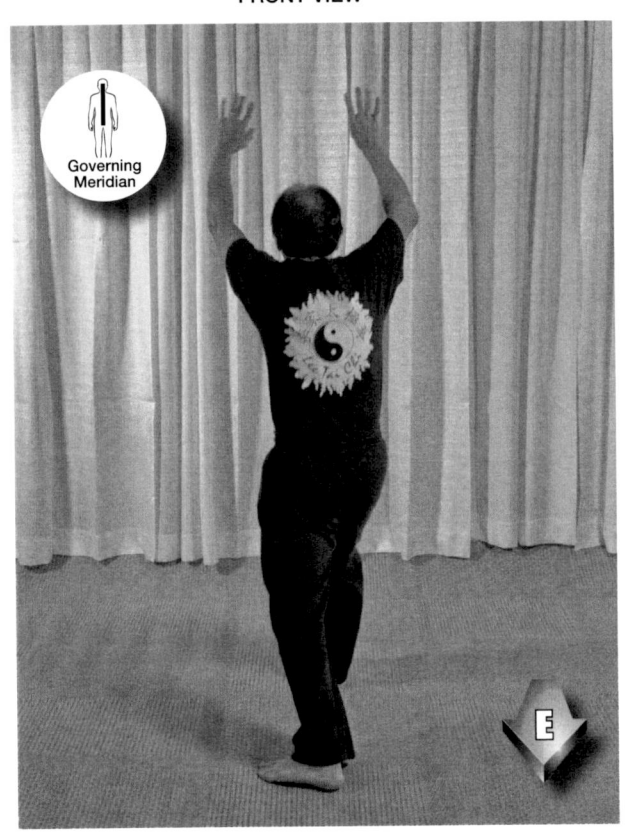

POSTURE 32-*INHALE*

Turn body 180° CW with hands extended out to the front, palms down. (Weight shifts from LF forward to RF forward as you turn) Finish by making CCW half circle with both arms, palms forward, ending with both hands out in front of body, above head.

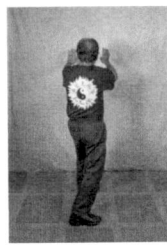

Sequential reverse view

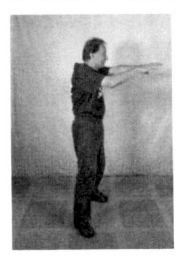

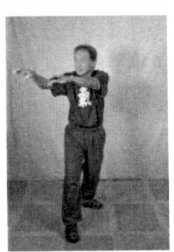

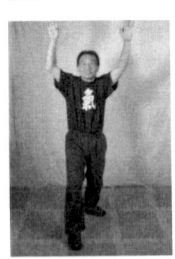

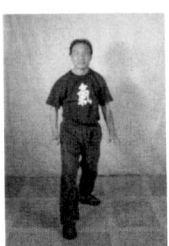

POSTURE 32-*EXHALE*

Hands move down to sides of body and slightly outward to each side. Palms face down.

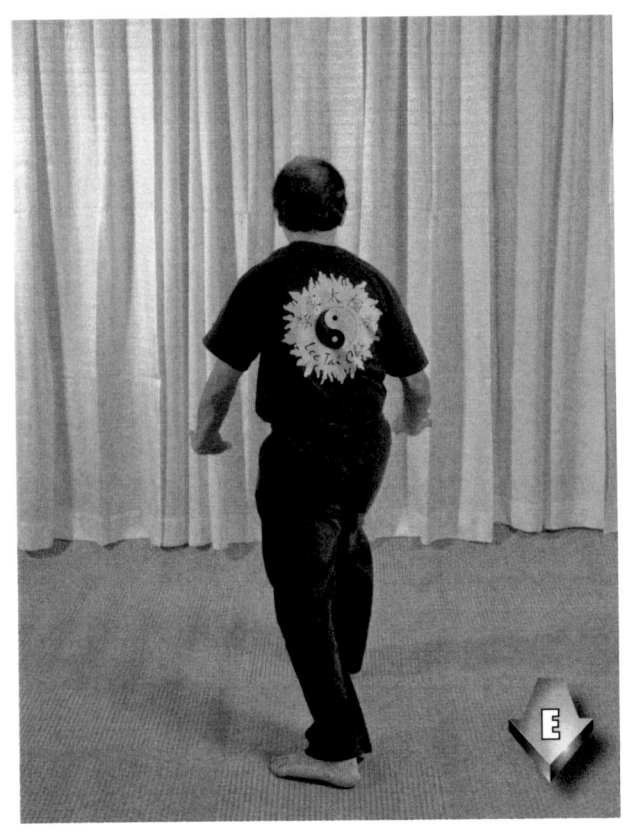

Posture 33

FRONT VIEW

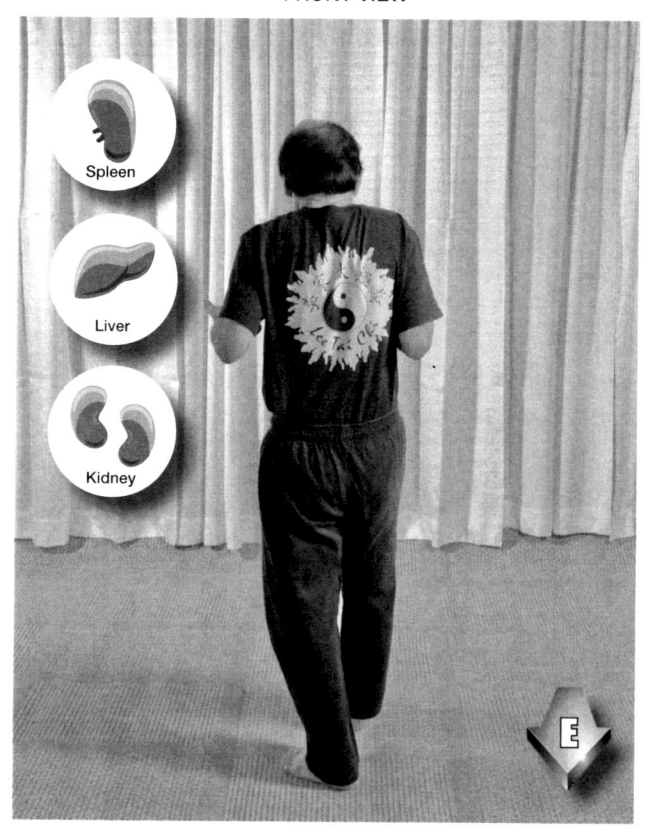

SIDE VIEW

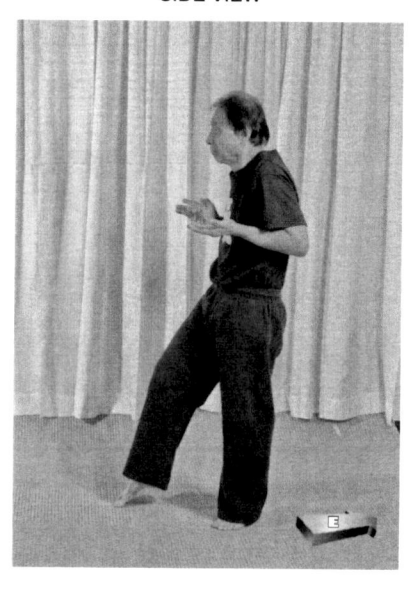

POSTURE 33-*INHALE*
Weight shifts to the rear leg as RF comes back to CS. Hands pull back to chest level.

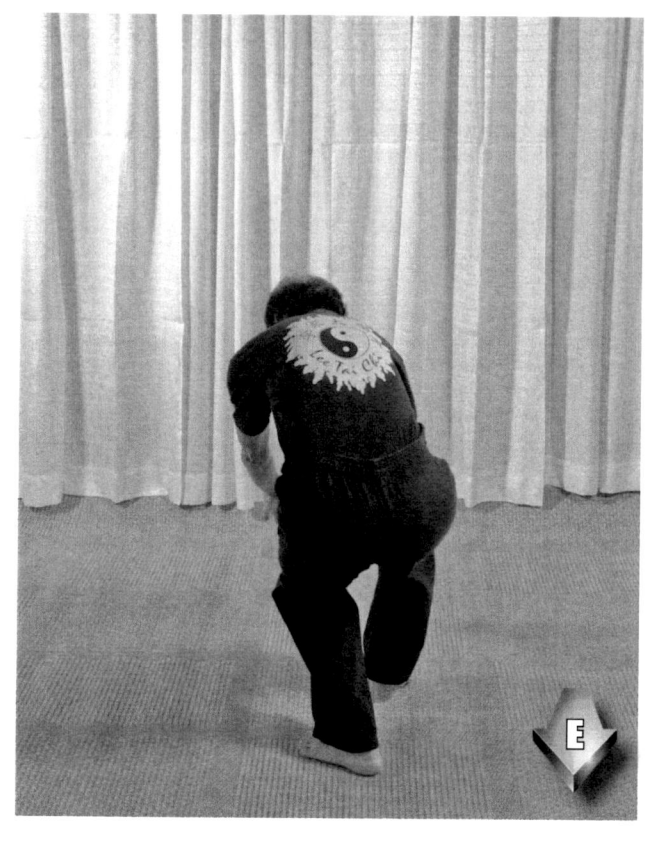

SIDE VIEW

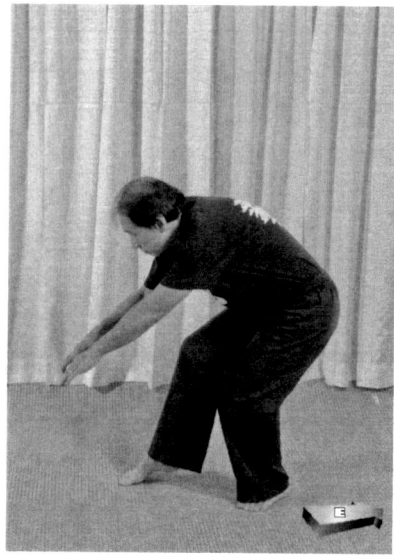

POSTURE 33-*EXHALE*
Hands rotate over to palm down as both hands extend down 45°, fingers pointing 45°.

Posture 34

FRONT VIEW

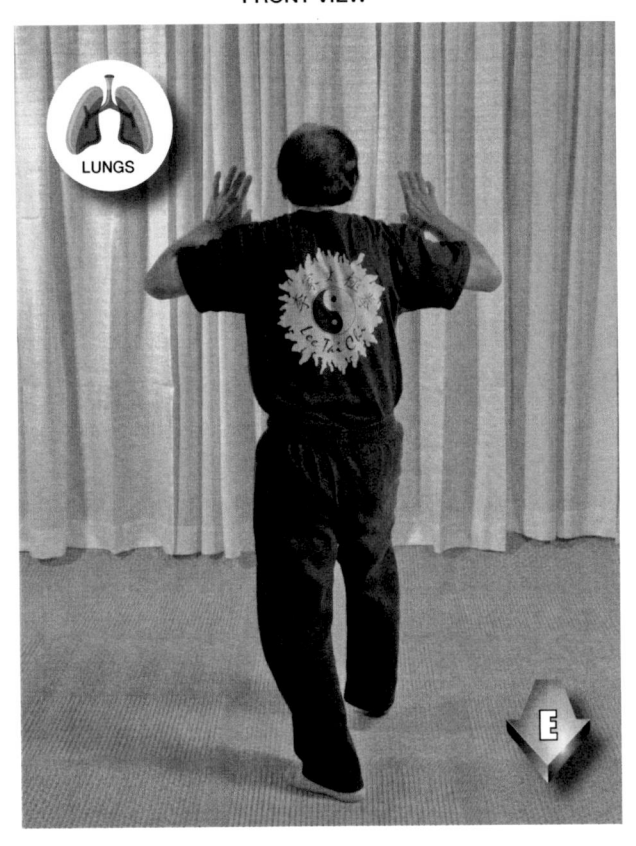

SIDE VIEW

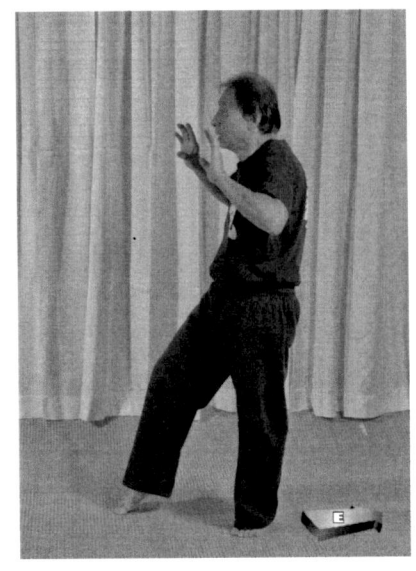

POSTURE 34-*INHALE*
Raise hands up in front, palms down, to shoulder height and then circle back towards the chest.

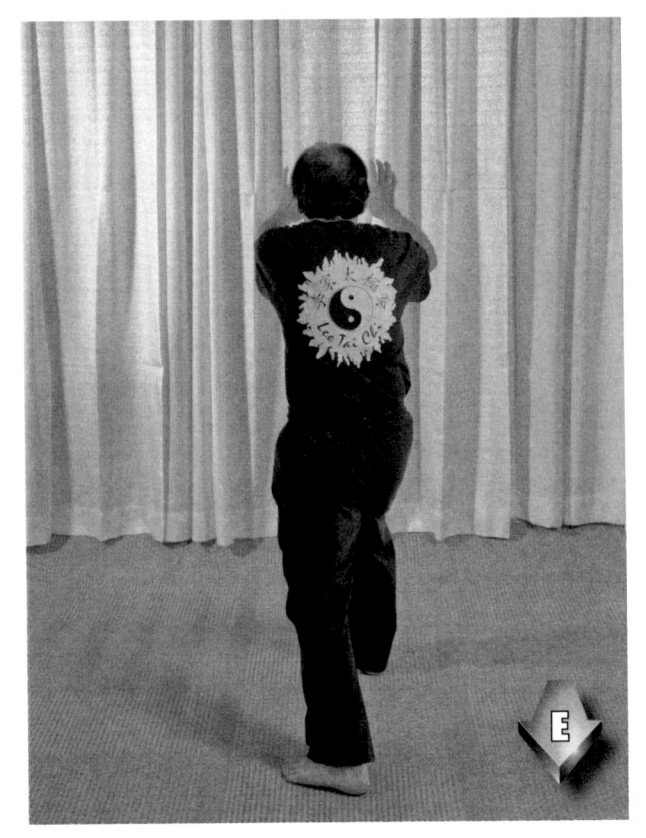

SIDE VIEW

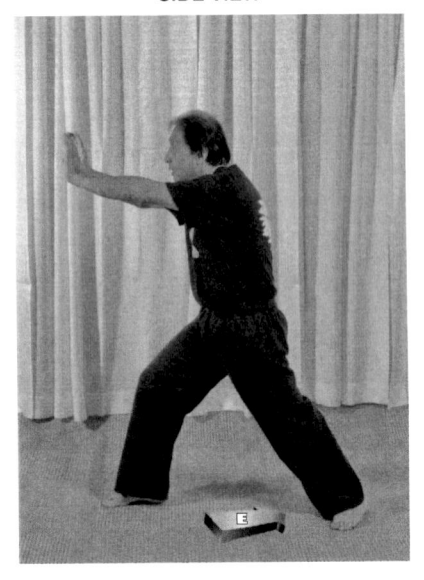

POSTURE 34-*EXHALE*
With palms facing forward, extend hands forward as RF steps into BS.

Posture 35

FRONT VIEW

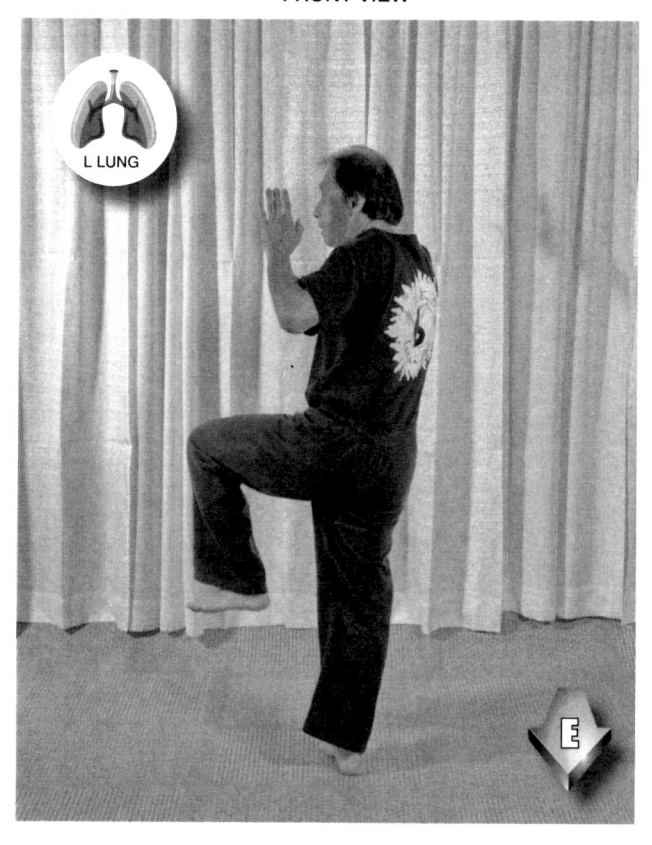

L LUNG

SIDE VIEW

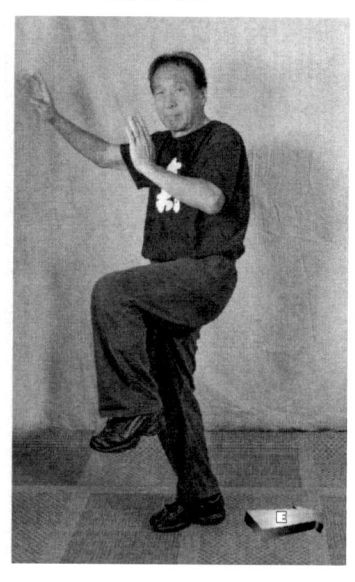

POSTURE 35-*INHALE*
LF raises as LH comes to left shoulder, then body turns to left. RH stays extended to front.

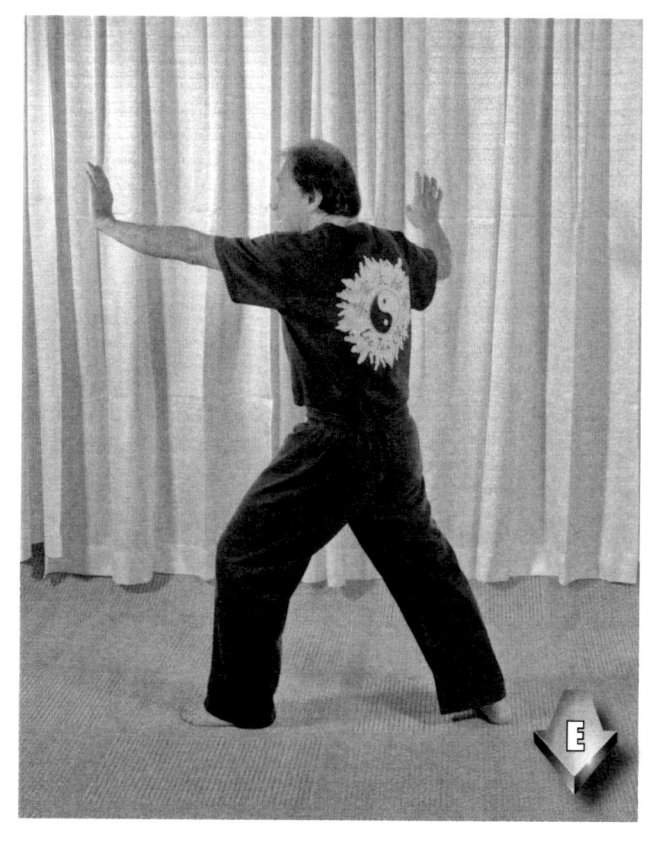

SIDE VIEW

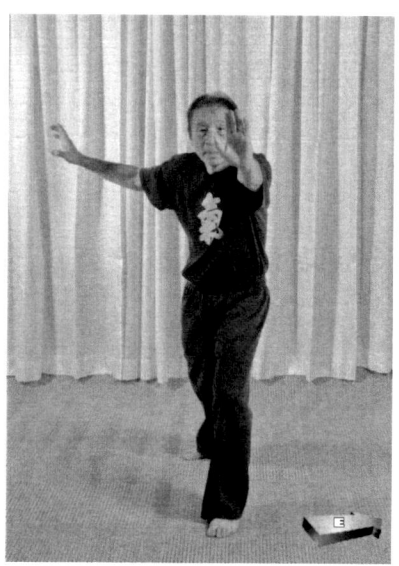

POSTURE 35-*EXHALE*
LF steps 90° to left and LH presses palm forward. RH stays in same position.

74

Posture 36

FRONT VIEW

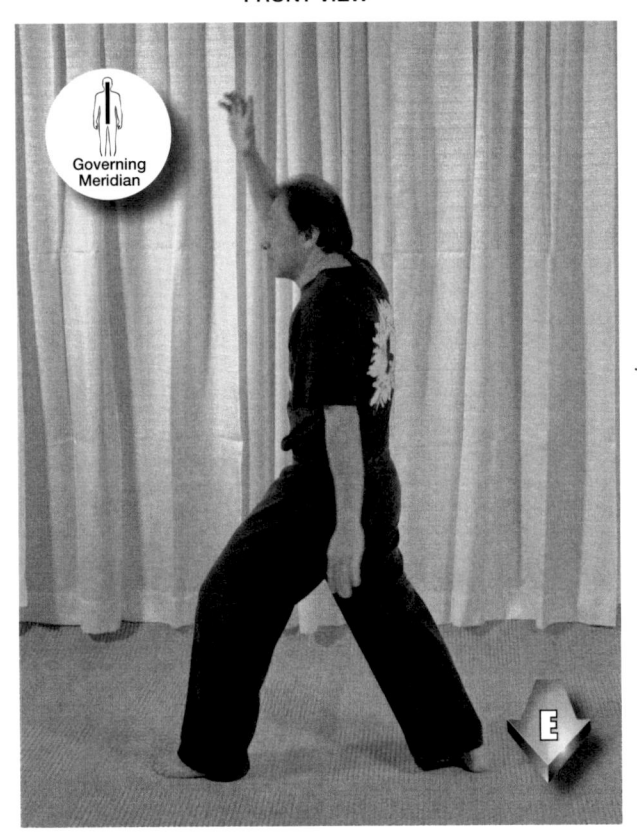

Governing Meridian

SIDE VIEW

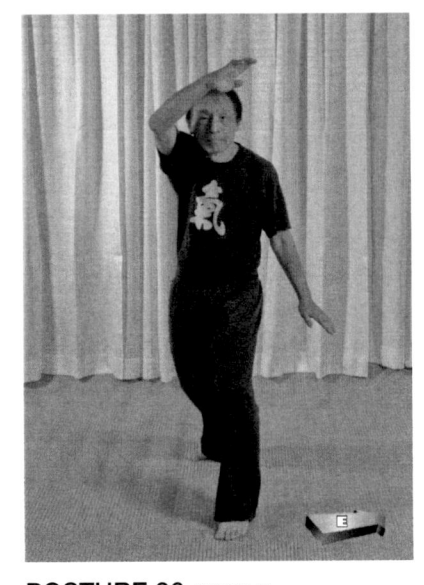

POSTURE 36-*INHALE*
RH circles up, then crosses in front of body as LH circles out to the left side.

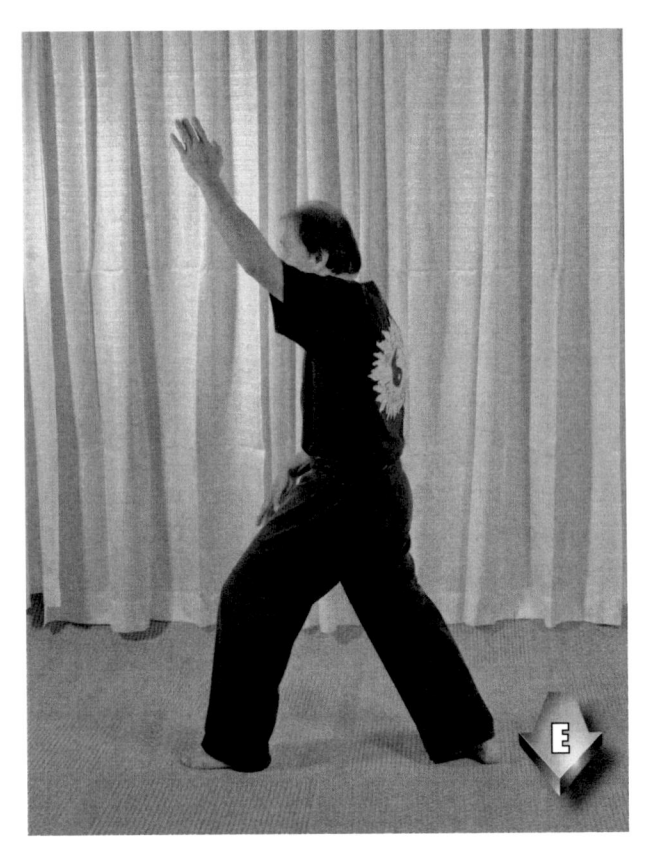

SIDE VIEW

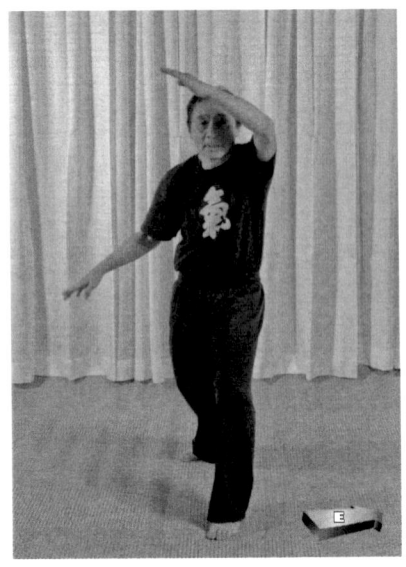

POSTURE 36-*EXHALE*
LH circles up and crosses in front of body as RH circles out to the right side.

Posture 37

FRONT VIEW

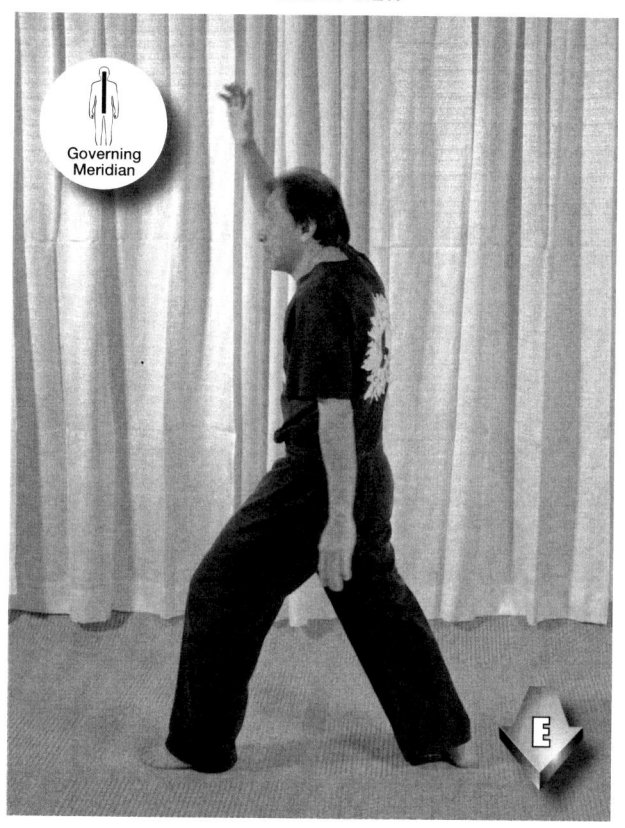

Governing Meridian

SIDE VIEW

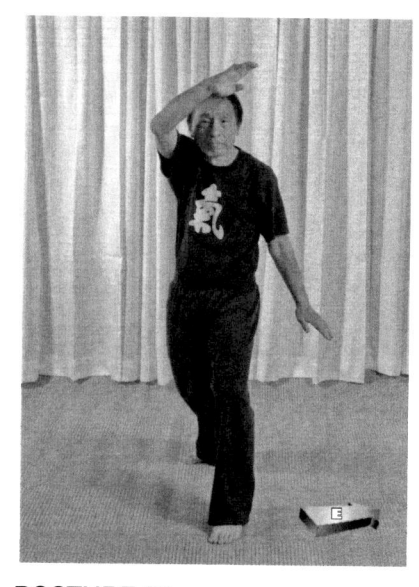

POSTURE 37-*INHALE*
RH circles up and crosses in front of body as LH circles out to the left side.

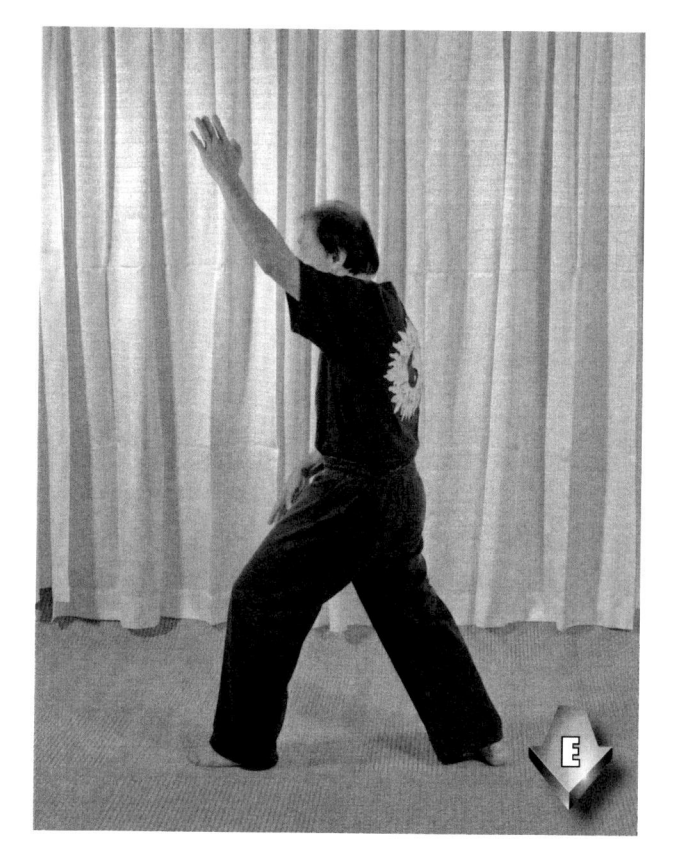

SIDE VIEW

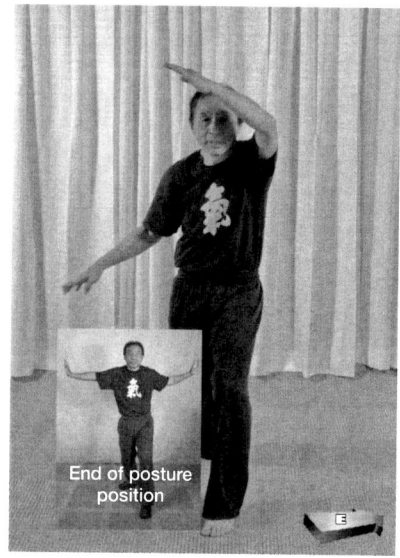

End of posture position

POSTURE 37-*EXHALE*
LH circles up and crosses in front of body as RH circles out to the right side. End posture with both arms out to the side and fingers up.

Posture 38

FRONT VIEW

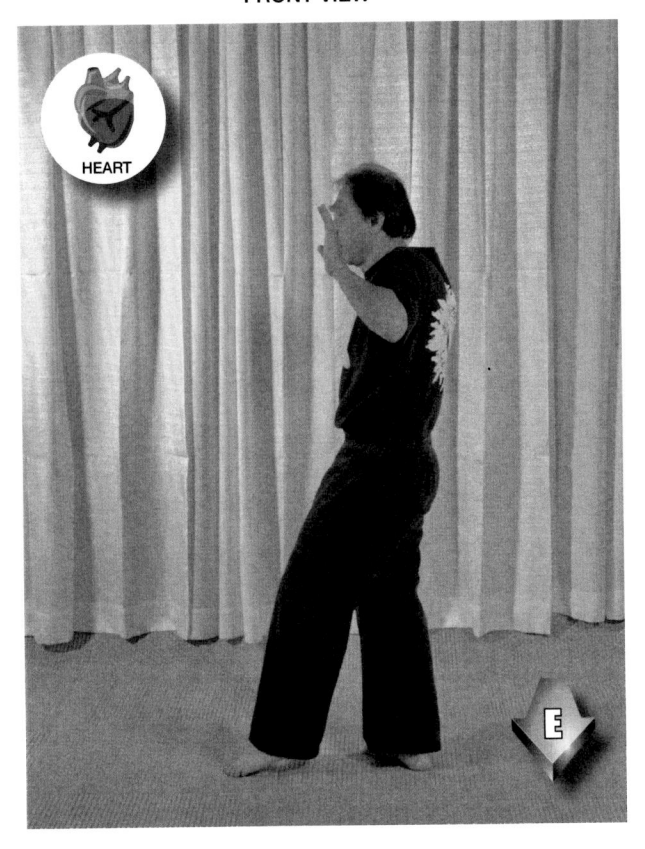

HEART

SIDE VIEW

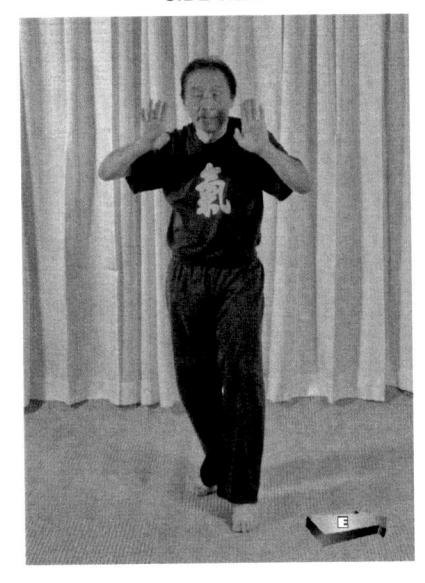

POSTURE 38-_INHALE_
Weight shifts to rear leg as LF comes back to CS and hands pull back to chest, palms forward..

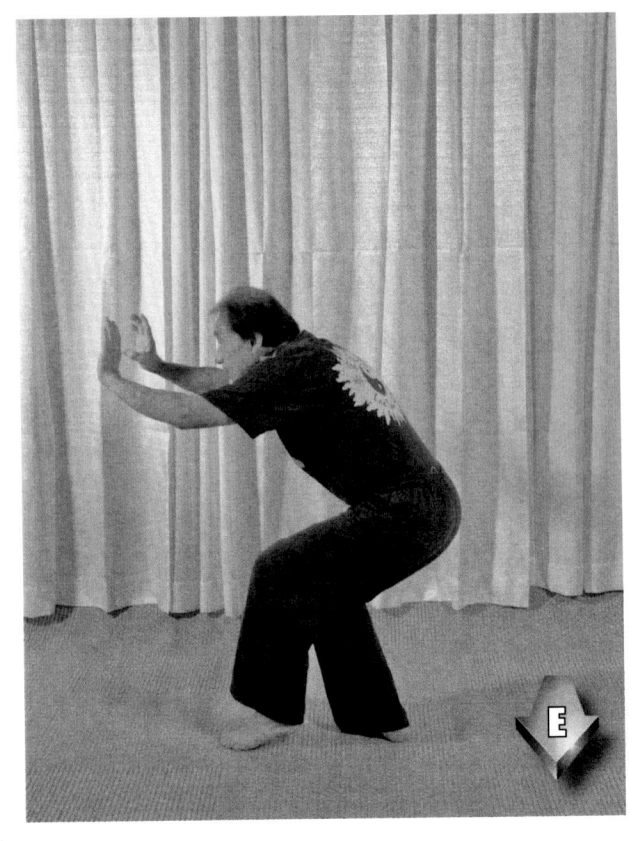

SIDE VIEW

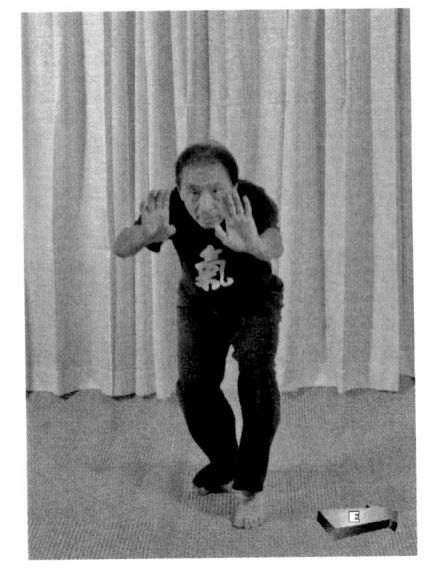

POSTURE 38-_EXHALE_
Hands extend forward and body sinks, bending at the knee

Posture 39

FRONT VIEW

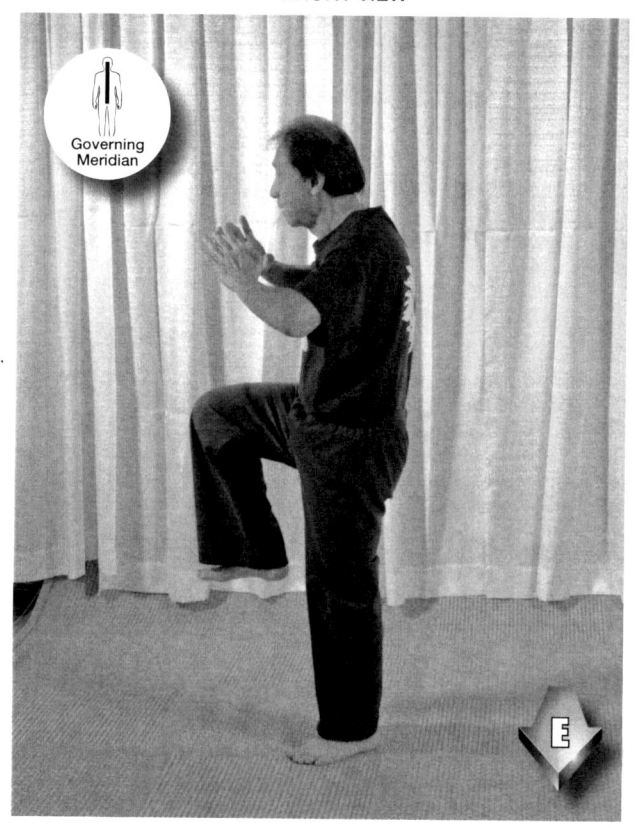

SIDE VIEW

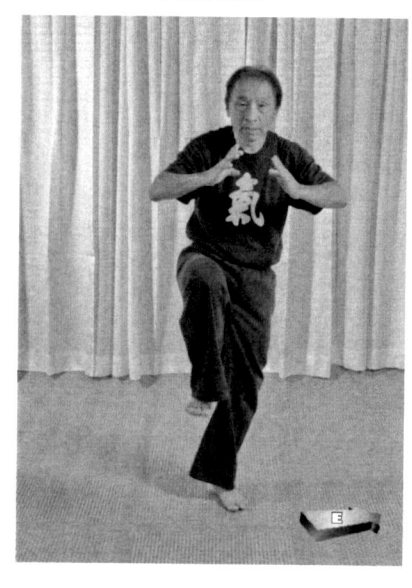

POSTURE 39-*INHALE*
Raise RF as body rises, hands turn fingers up, palms facing each other at chest level.

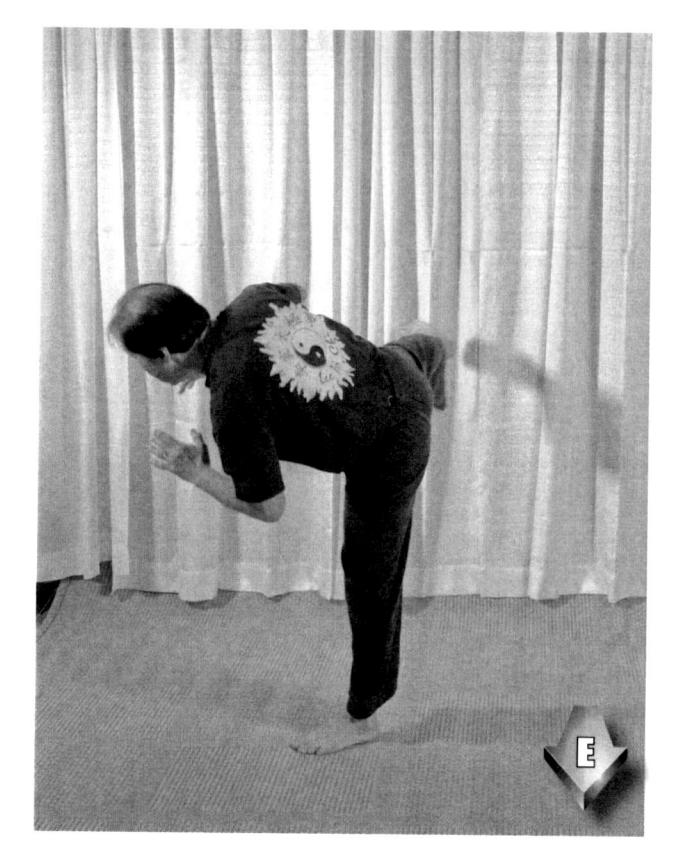

SIDE VIEW

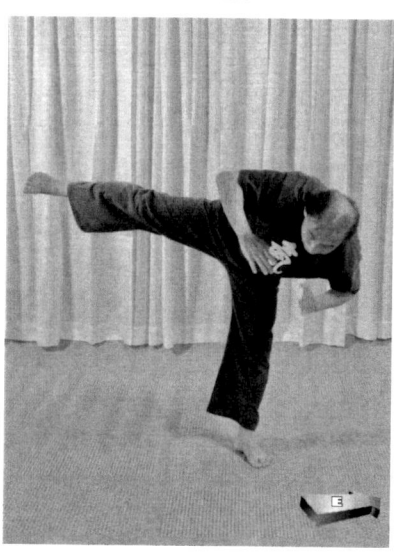

POSTURE 39-*EXHALE*
Extend RF out to right side as upper body leans to left.

Posture 40

FRONT VIEW

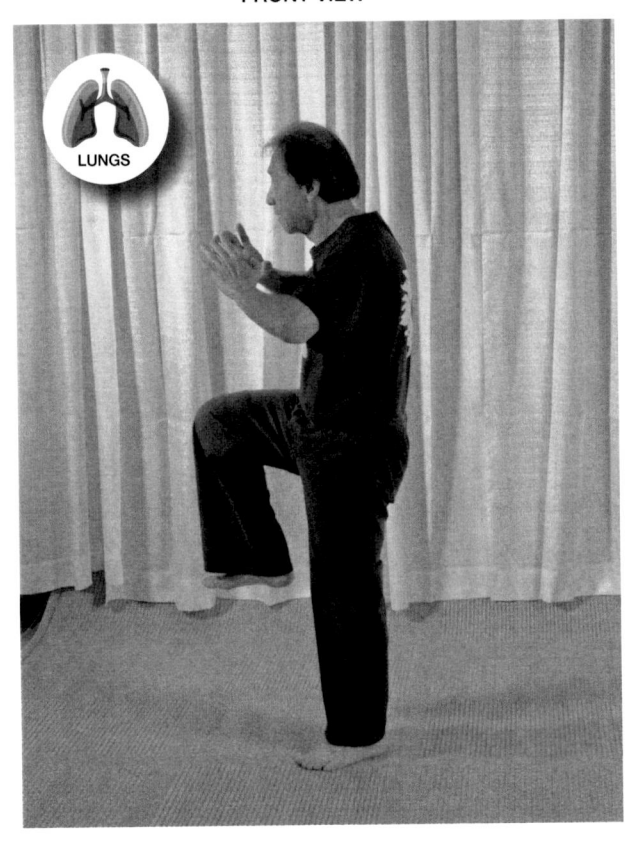

LUNGS

SIDE VIEW

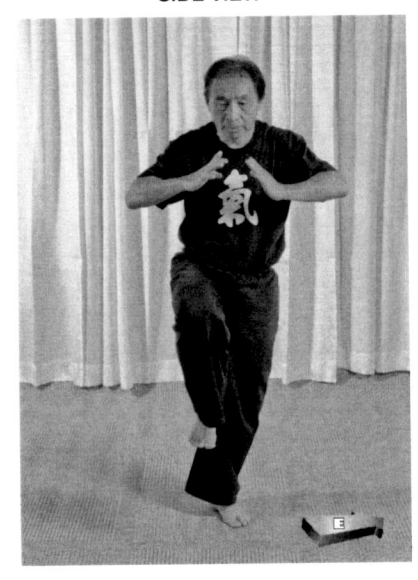

POSTURE 40-*INHALE*
RF comes back in as body goes back to vertical with hands front of the chest

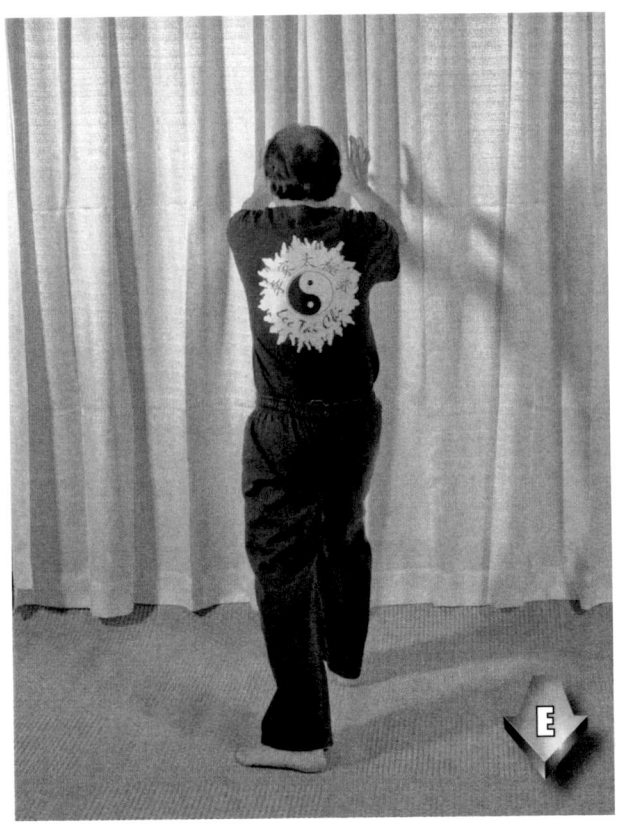

SIDE VIEW

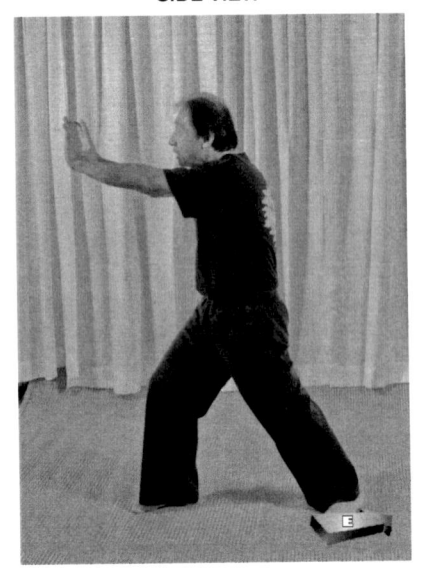

POSTURE 40-*EXHALE*
Body rotates to right on left leg. RF steps out into BS and hands extend to the front, palms facing forward

Posture 41

FRONT VIEW

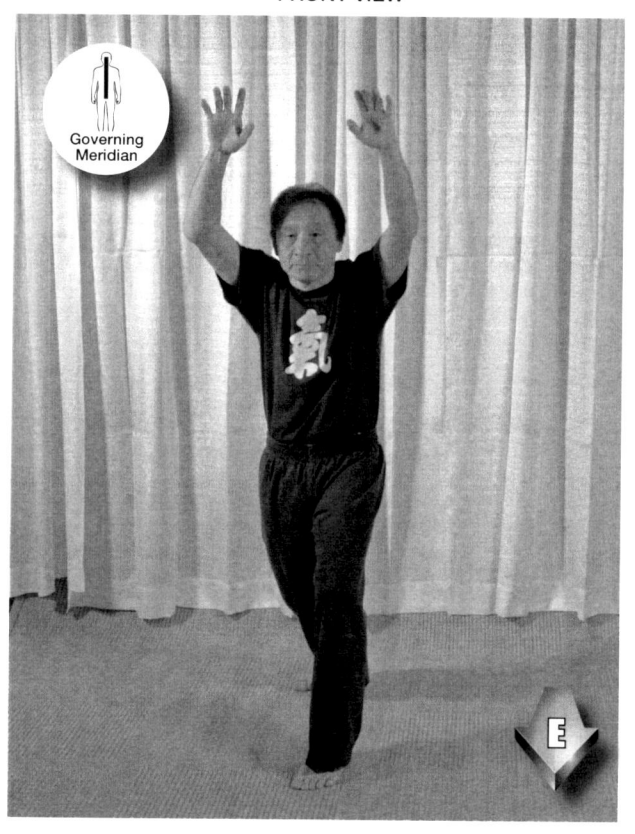

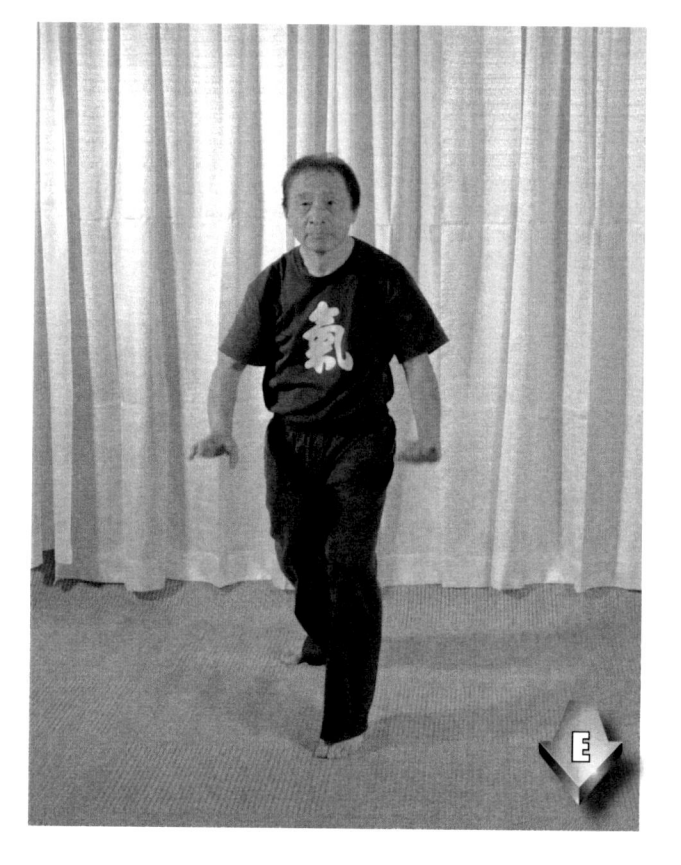

POSTURE 41 -*INHALE*

Turn body 180° CCW with hands extended out to the front, palms down. (Weight shifts from RF forward to LF forward as you turn) Finish by making CW half circle with both arms, palms forward, ending with both hands out in front of body, above head, palms down.

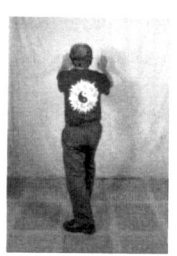

Sequential view

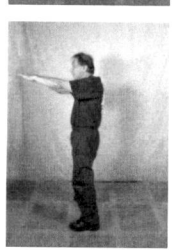

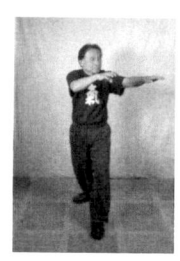

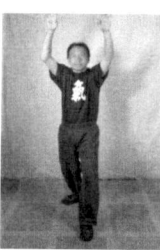

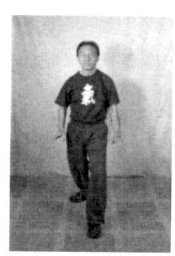

POSTURE 41 -*EXHALE*

Hands drop down to sides of body and slightly outward to each side.

Posture 42

FRONT VIEW

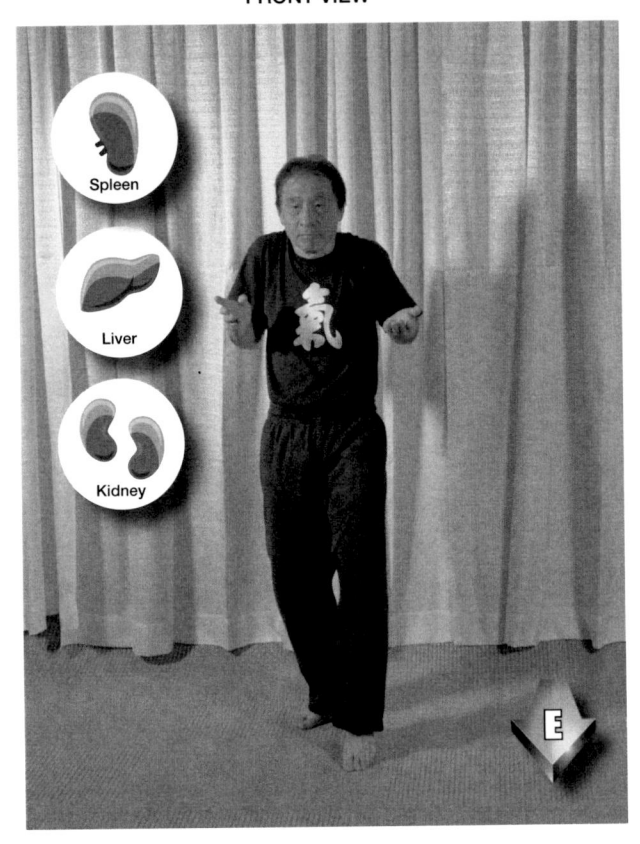

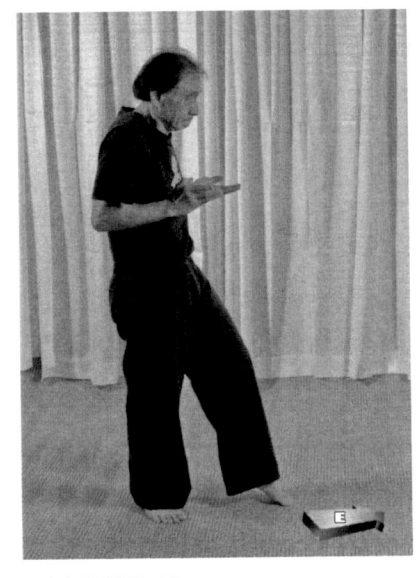

POSTURE 42-INHALE
Weight shifts to rear leg as LF comes back to CS. Hands pull back at chest level.

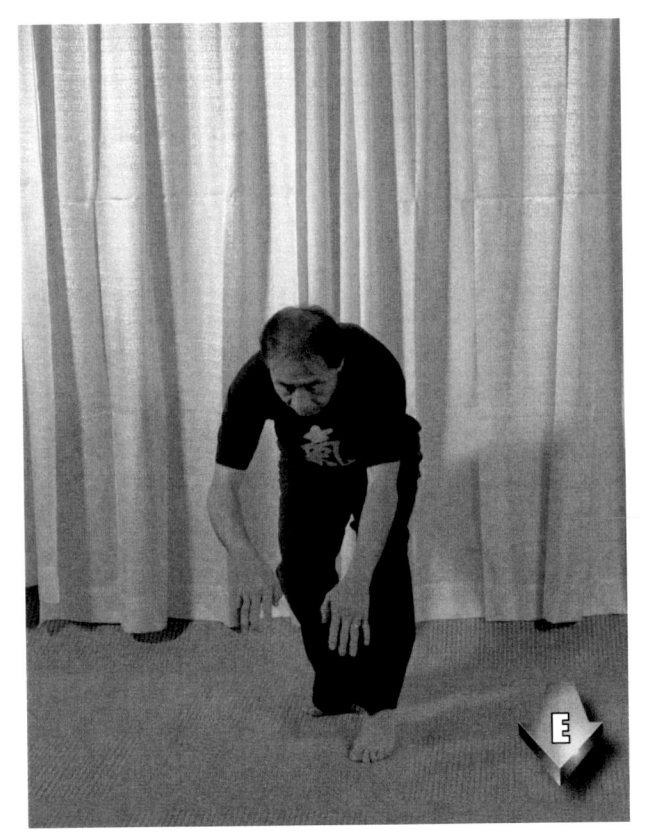

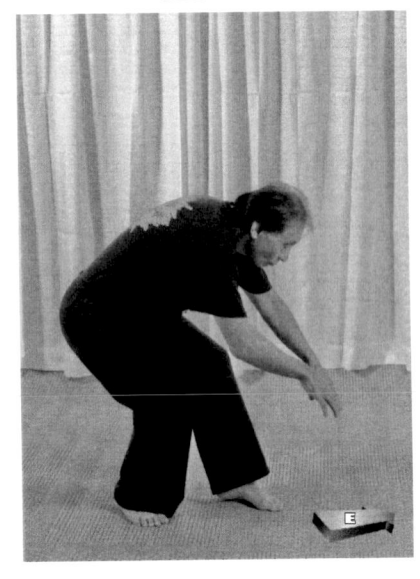

POSTURE 42-EXHALE
Hands rotate over to palm down as both hands extend down 45°, fingers pointing down 45°.

Posture 43

FRONT VIEW

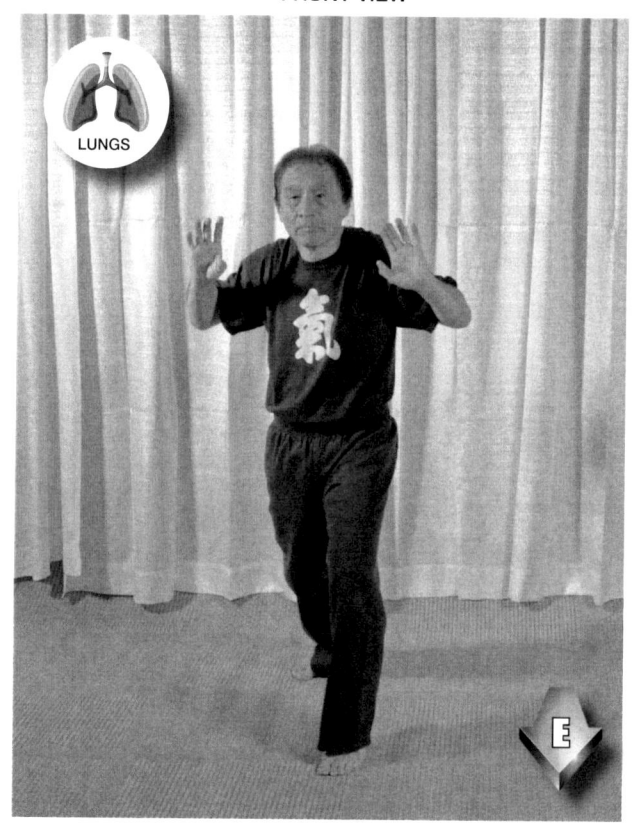

SIDE VIEW

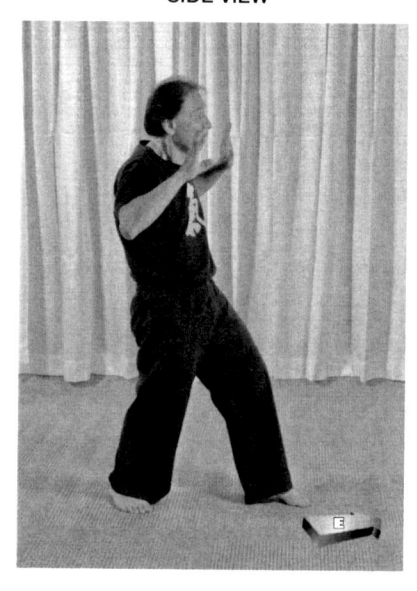

POSTURE 43-*INHALE*
Raise hands up in front, palms down, to shoulder height and then circle back towards chest, ending palms facing forward.

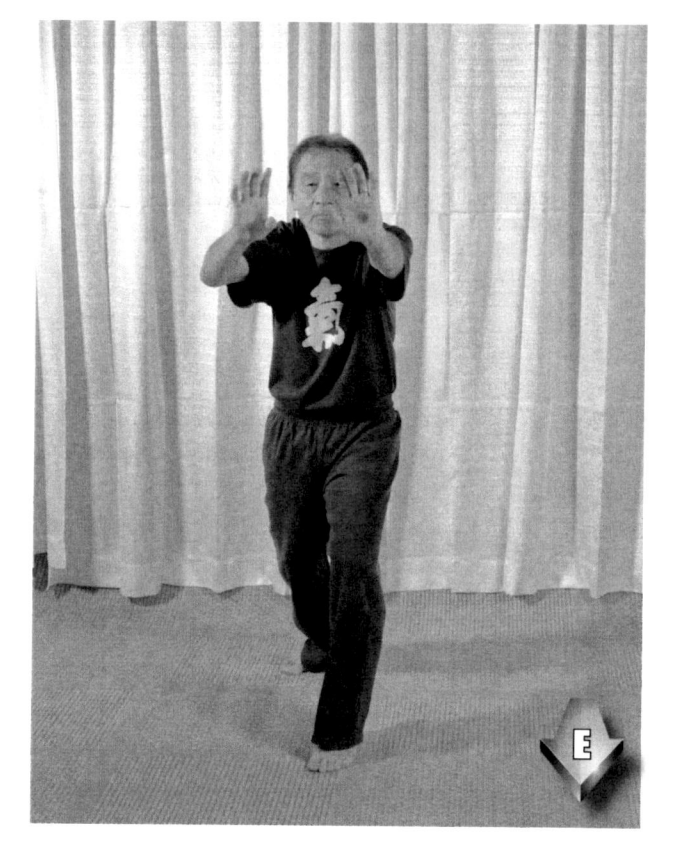

SIDE VIEW

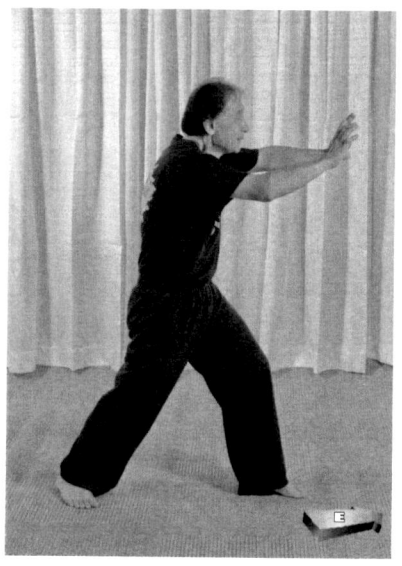

POSTURE 43-*EXHALE*
With palms facing forward, extend hands forward as LF steps into BS.

Posture 44

FRONT VIEW

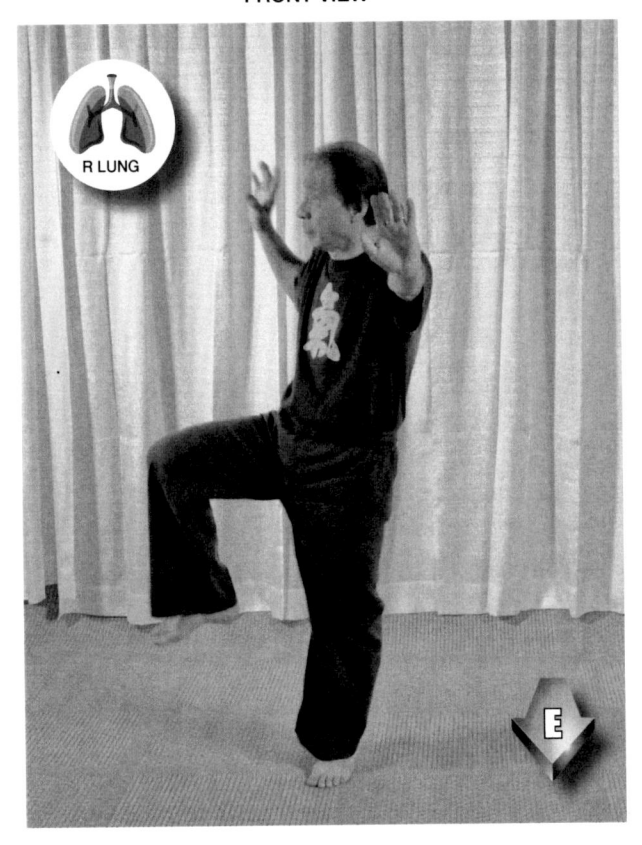

R LUNG

SIDE VIEW

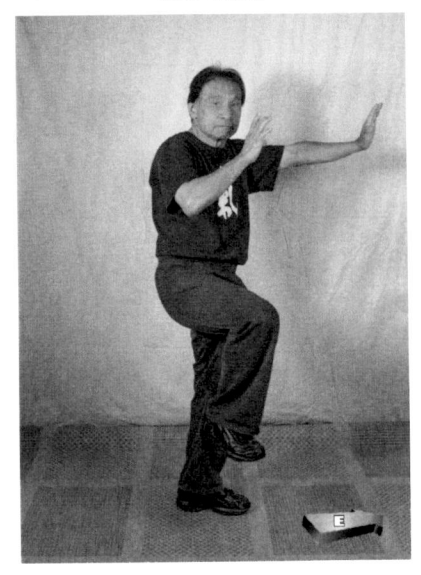

POSTURE 44-*INHALE*
RF raises as RH comes to right shoulder, then body rotates to right. LH stays extended to front.

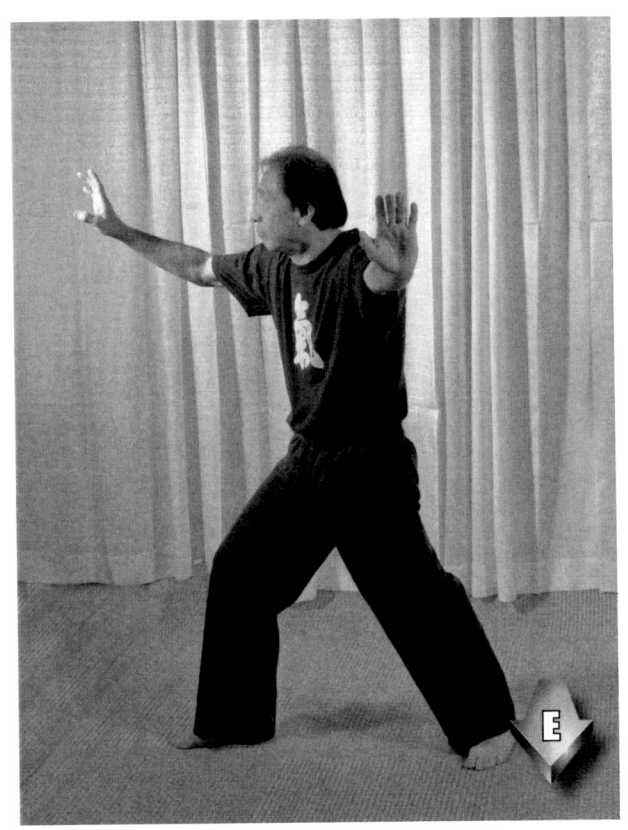

SIDE VIEW

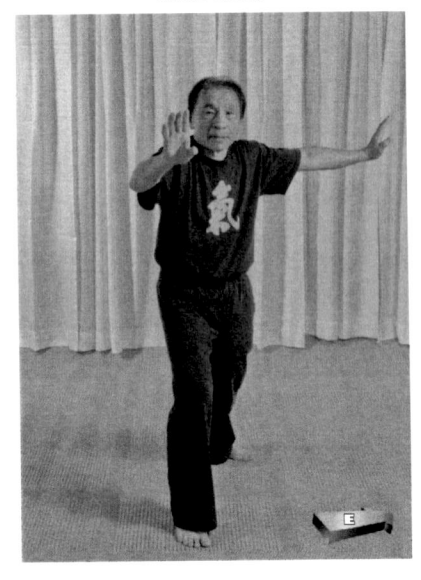

POSTURE 44-*EXHALE*
RF steps 90° to right and RH presses palm forward. LH stays in same position.

Posture 45

FRONT VIEW

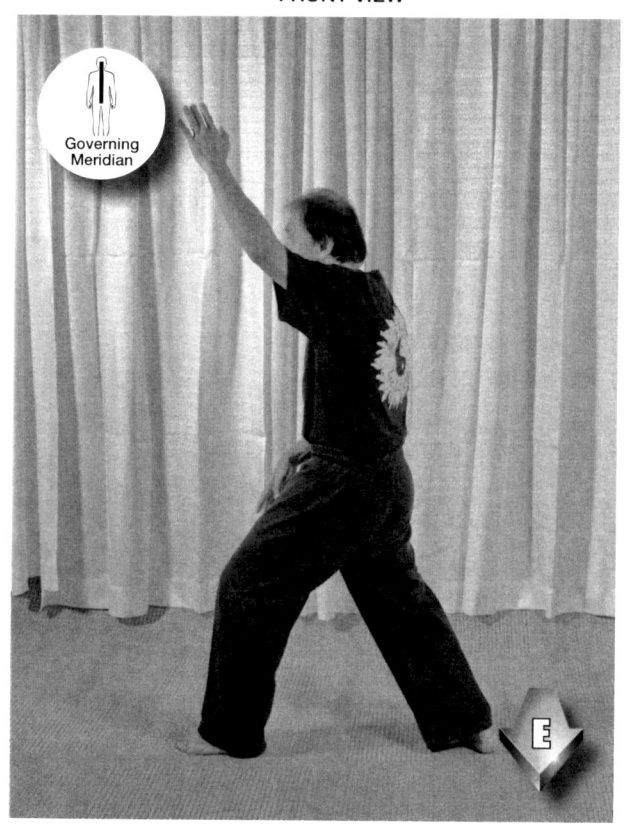

SIDE VIEW

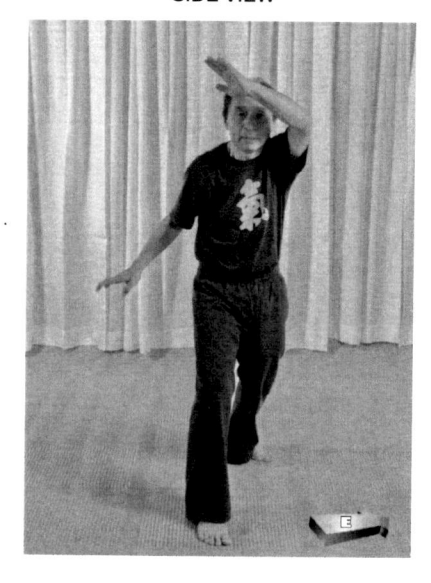

Governing Meridian

POSTURE 45-*INHALE*
LH circles up and then crosses in front of body as RH circles out to the left side.

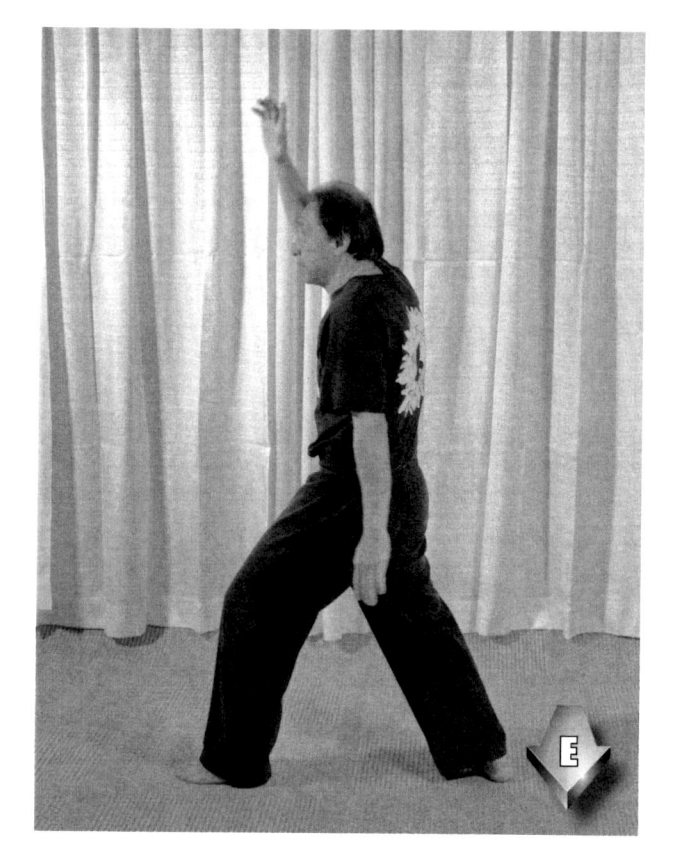

SIDE VIEW

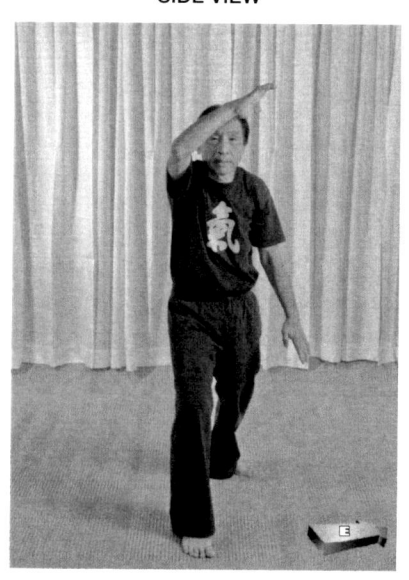

POSTURE 45-*EXHALE*
RH circles up and then crosses in front of body as LH circles out to the right side.

Posture 46

FRONT VIEW

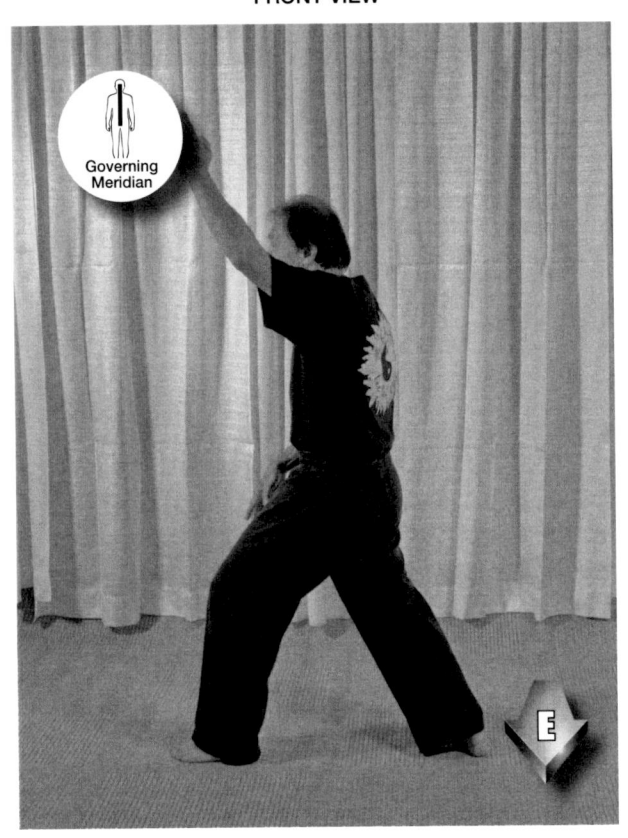

SIDE VIEW

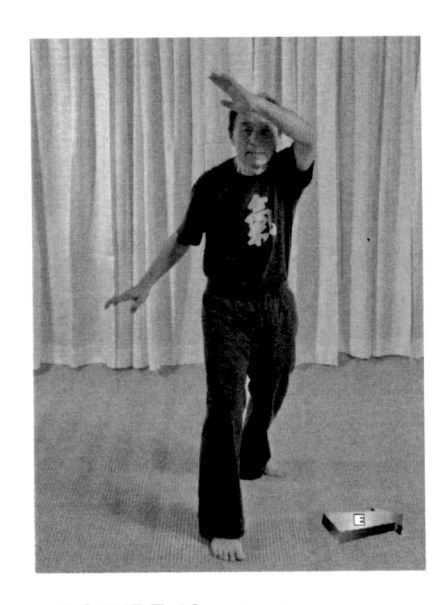

POSTURE 46-*INHALE*
LH circles up and then crosses in front of body as RH circles out to the left side.

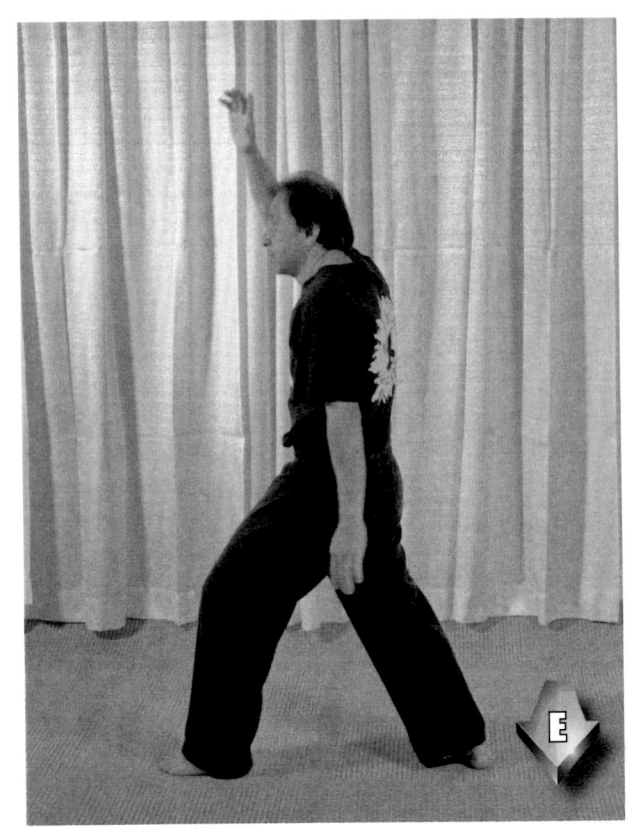

SIDE VIEW

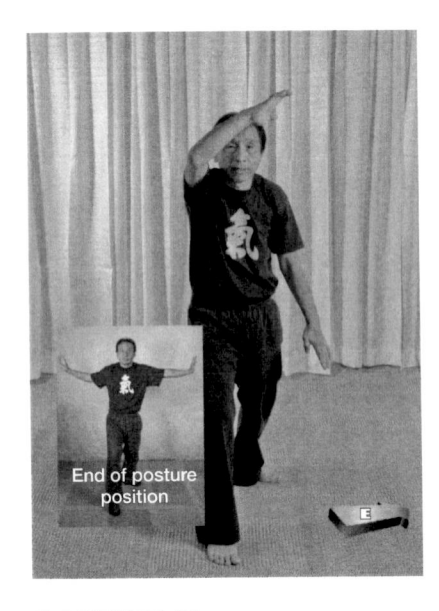

POSTURE 46-*EXHALE*
RH crosses in front of body as LH circles out to the left side. End posture with both arms out to the side and fingers pointing up.

Posture 47

FRONT VIEW

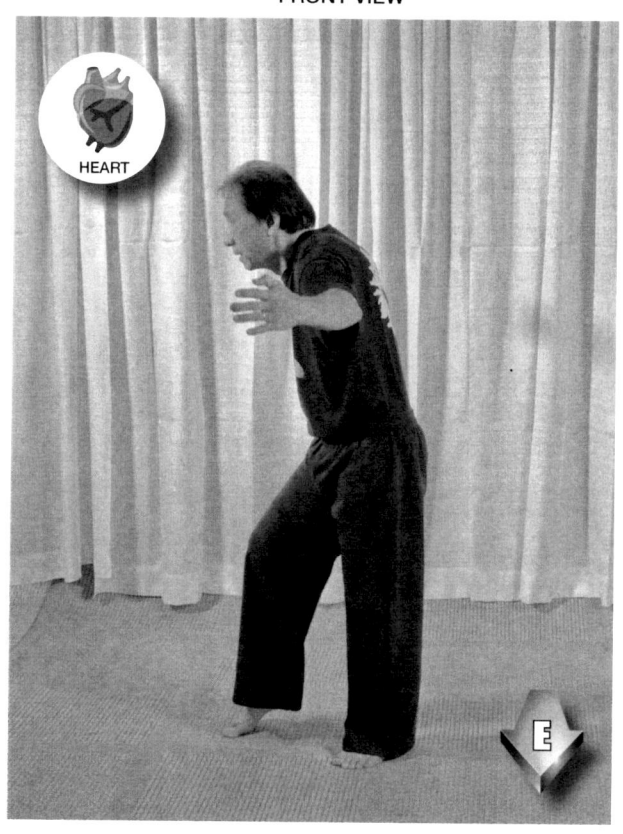

SIDE VIEW

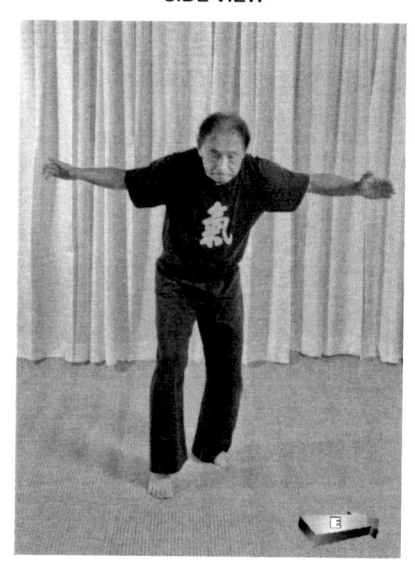

POSTURE 47-INHALE
RF moves back to CS as hands are extended out at shoulder level, palms forward.

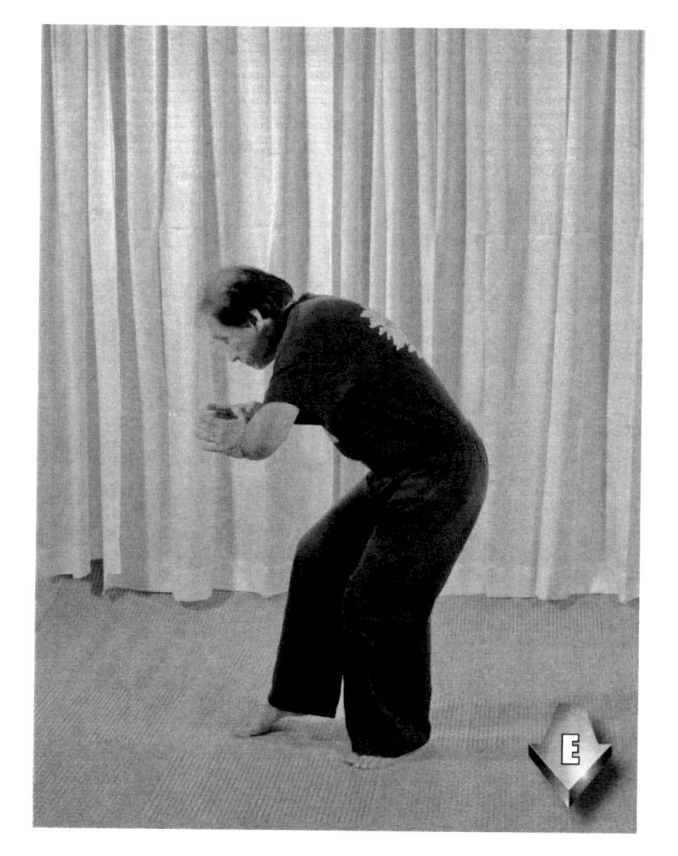

SIDE VIEW

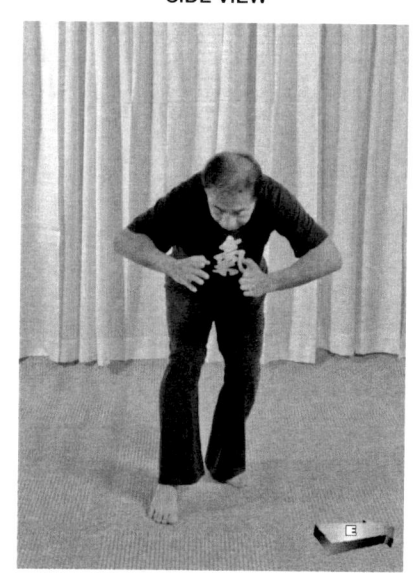

POSTURE 47-EXHALE
Hands press palms together with fingers pointing to the front (elbows up) and body sinks, bending at the knee.

Posture 48

FRONT VIEW

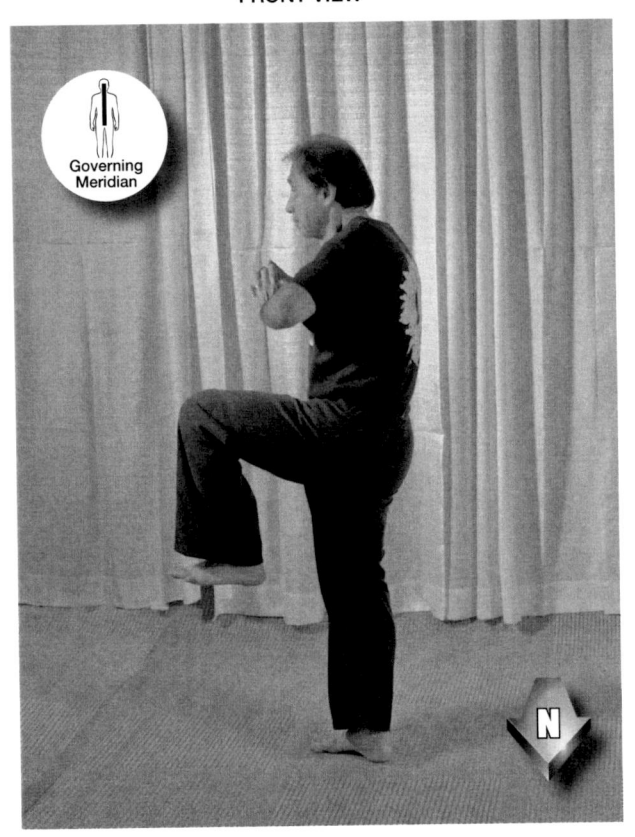

Governing Meridian

SIDE VIEW

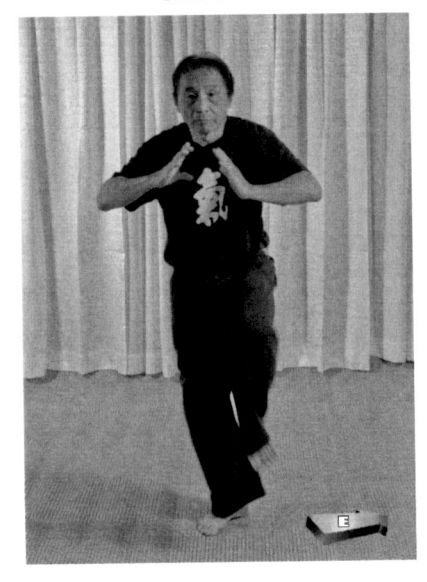

POSTURE 48-*INHALE*
Raise LF as body rises, hands turn fingers up, palms facing each other at chest level.

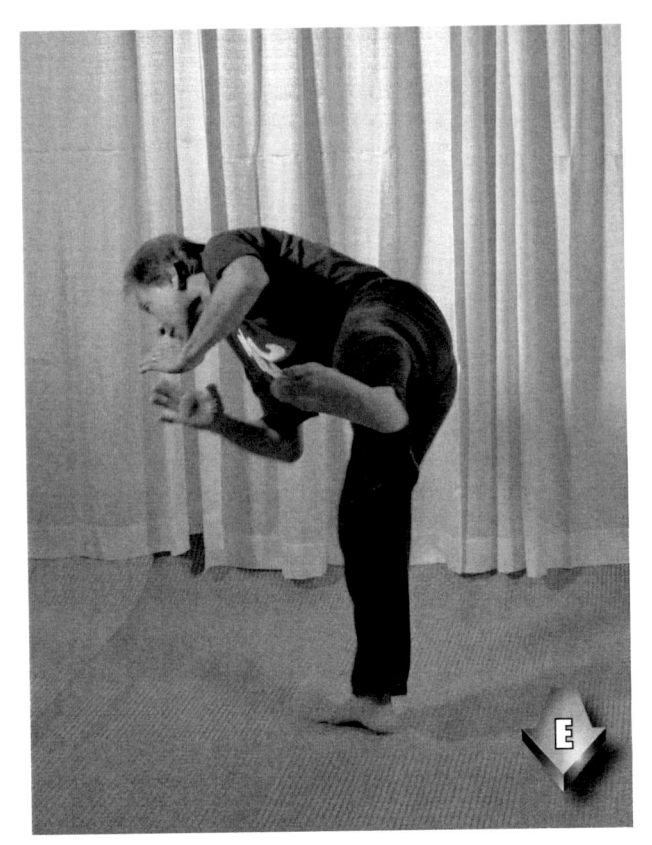

SIDE VIEW

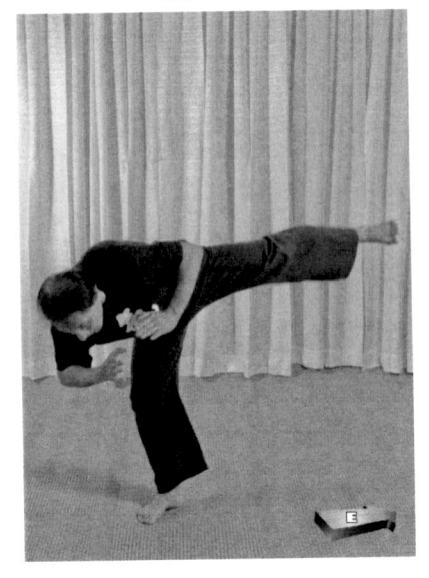

POSTURE 48-*EXHALE*
Extend LF out to left side as upper body leans to right.

Posture 49

FRONT VIEW

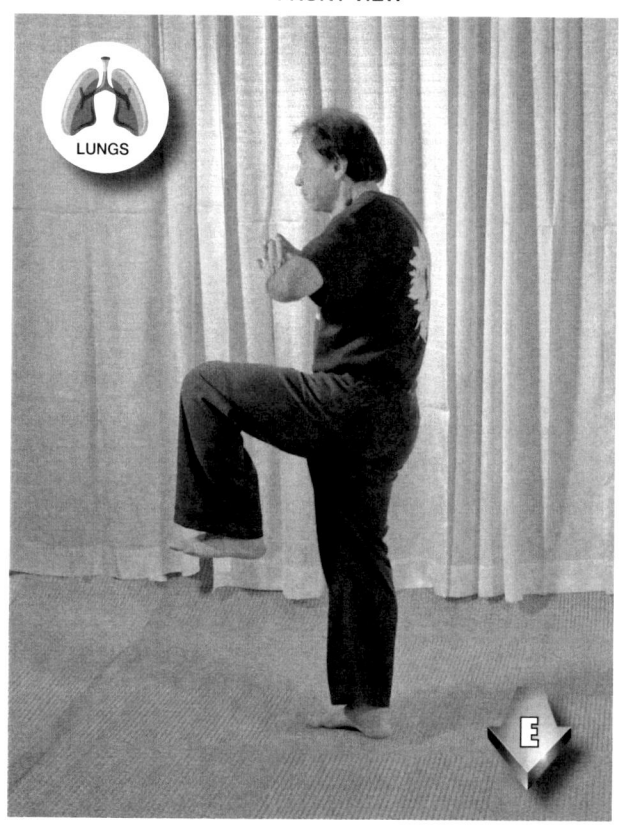

SIDE VIEW

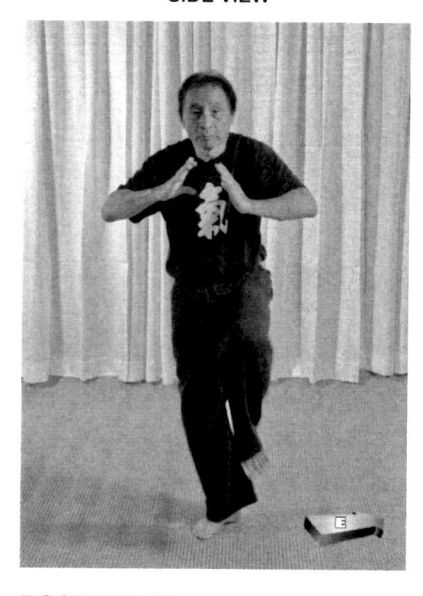

POSTURE 49-*INHALE*
LF comes back in as body goes back to vertical with hands front of the chest.

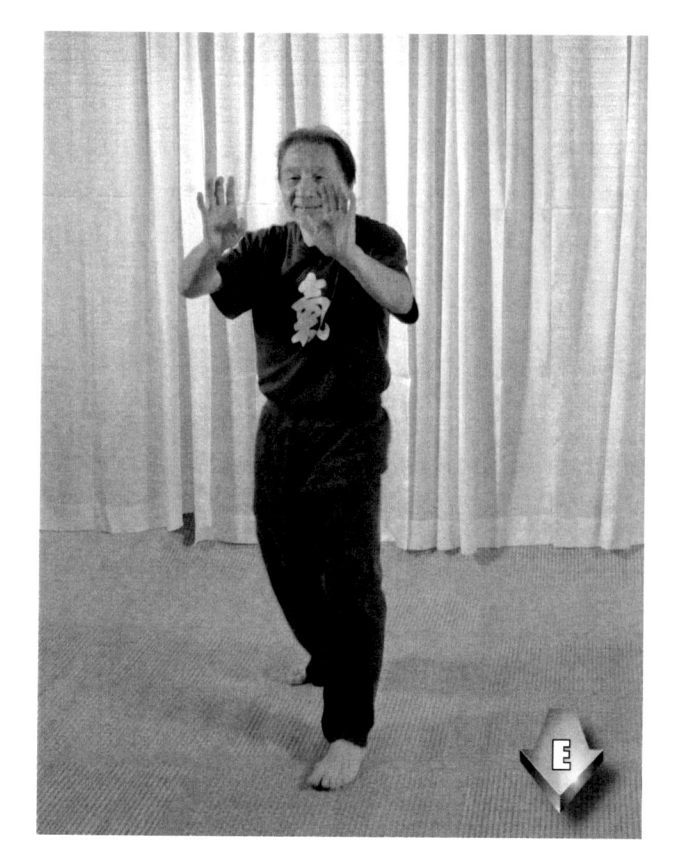

SIDE VIEW

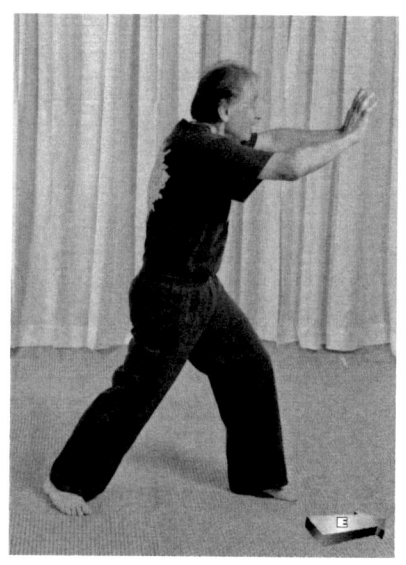

POSTURE 49-*EXHALE*
Body rotates to left on right leg. LF steps out into BS and hands extend to the front, palms facing forward.

Posture 50

FRONT VIEW

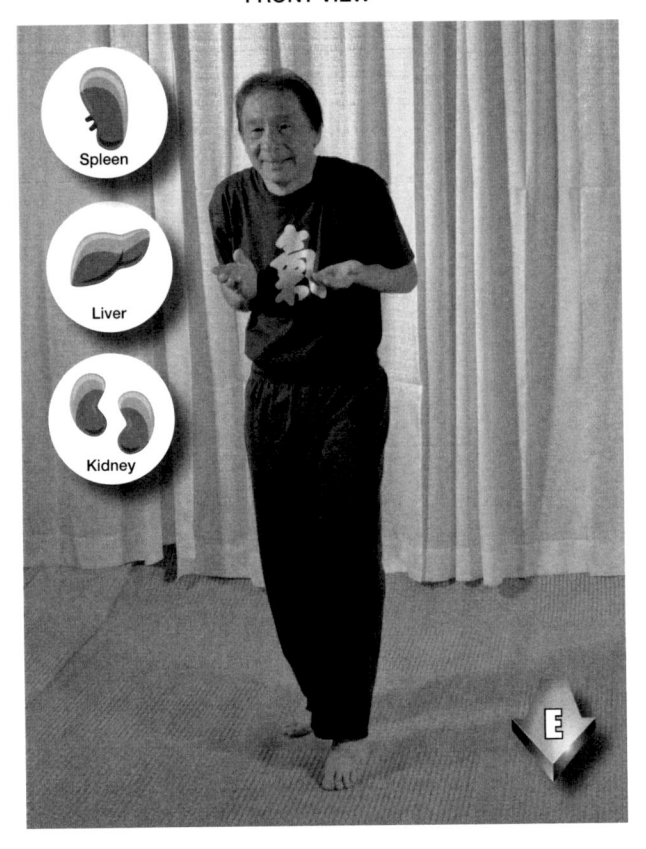

SIDE VIEW

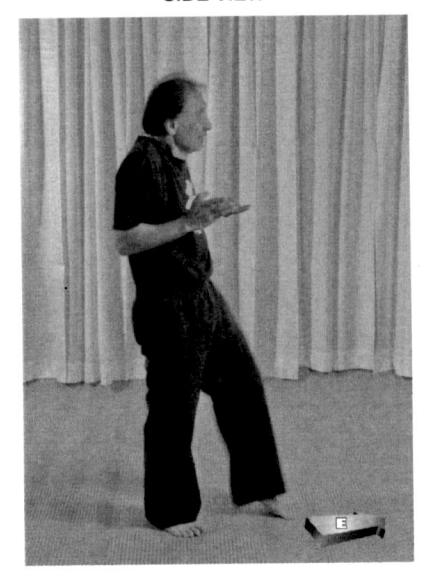

POSTURE 50-_INHALE_
Weight shifts to RF as both hands circle up and out to the side, as LF moves back to CS. Hands continue inward to chest level, palms up..

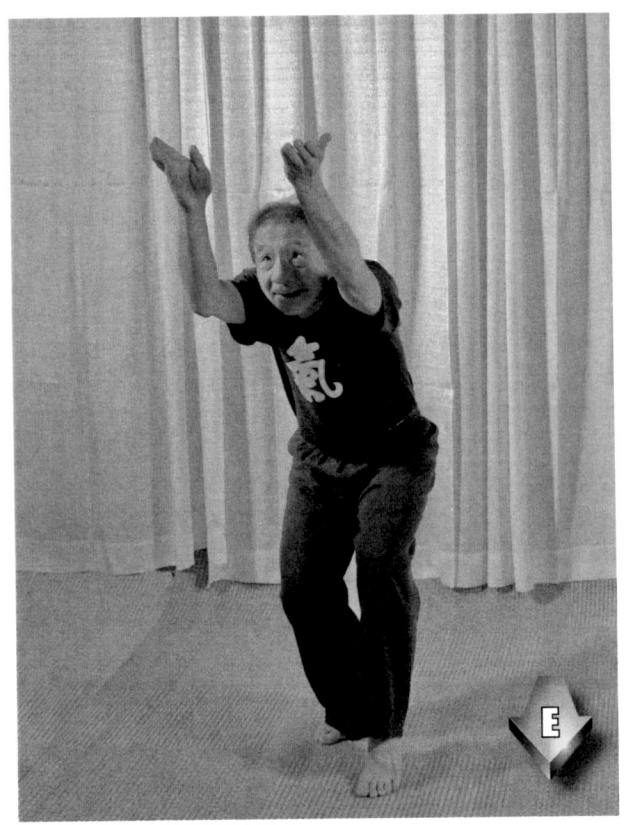

SIDE VIEW

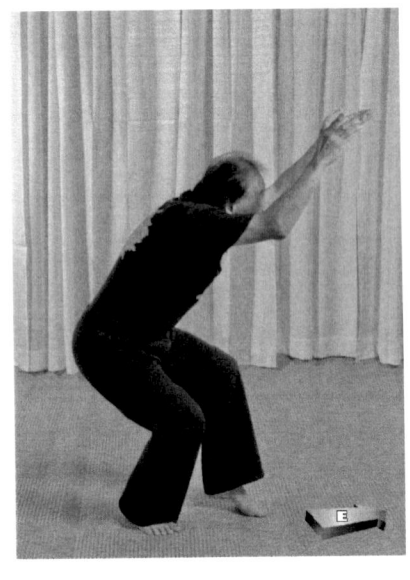

POSTURE 50-_EXHALE_
As you sink your stance, arms extend up above head with palms facing up.

Posture 51

FRONT VIEW

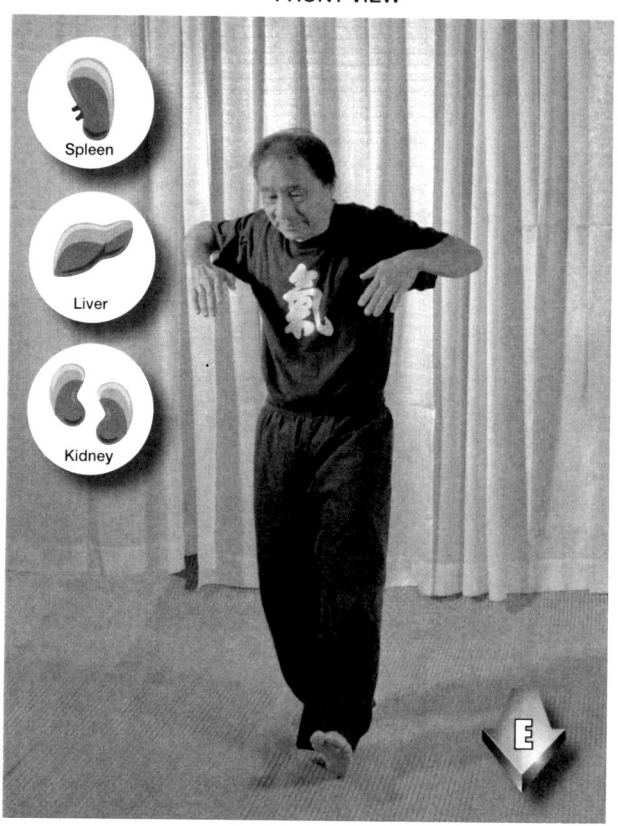

SIDE VIEW

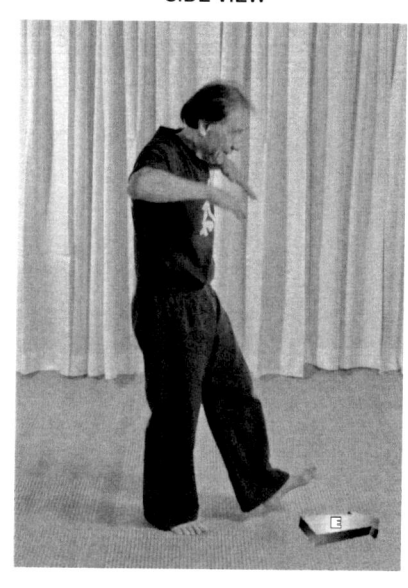

POSTURE 51-*INHALE*
LF moves to a heel stance as you rotate hands palms down and bring them in to the body, chest level.

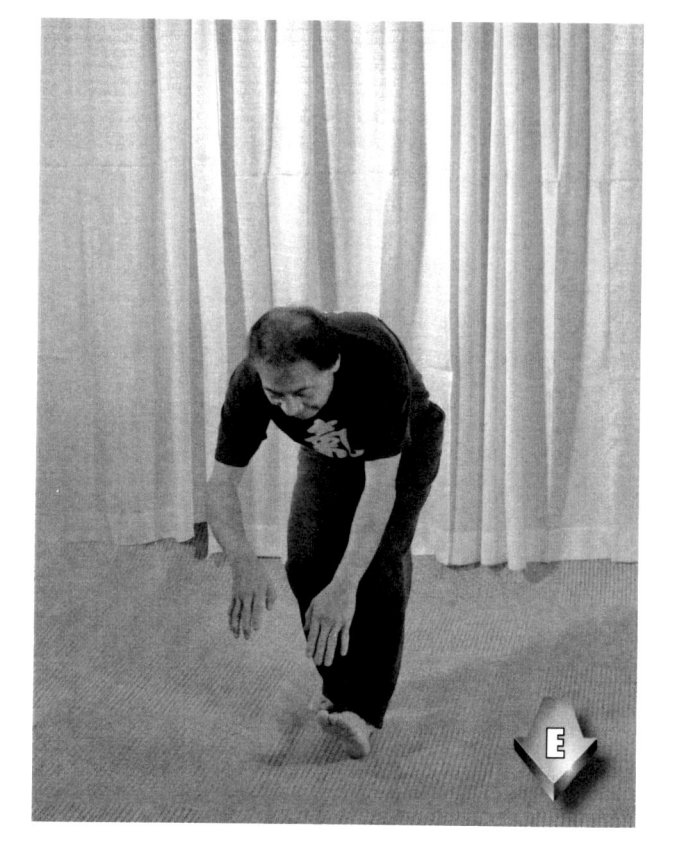

SIDE VIEW

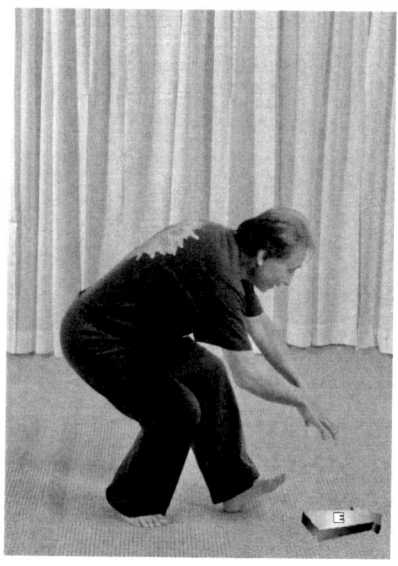

POSTURE 52-*EXHALE*
Hands extend down with fingertips 45° in front of the body as stance sinks.

Posture 52

FRONT VIEW

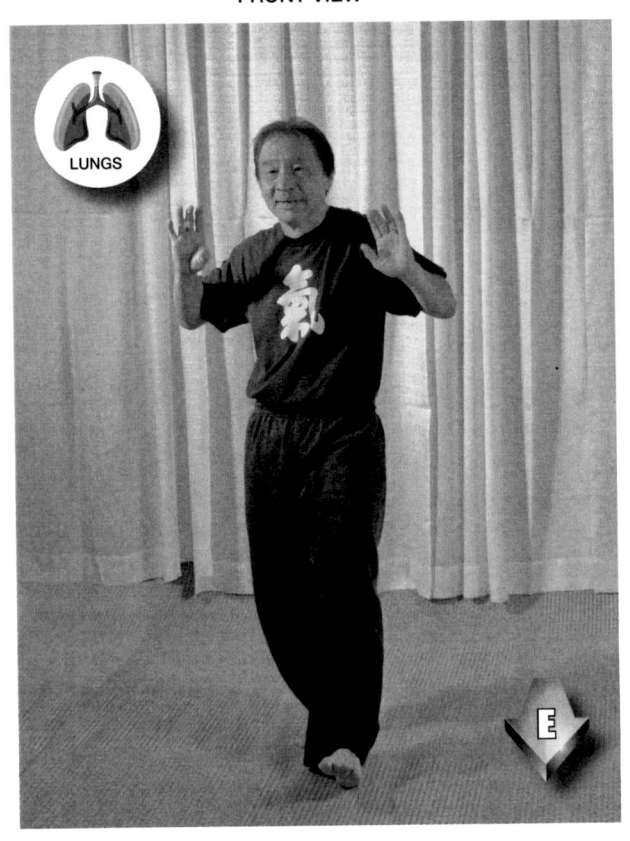

SIDE VIEW

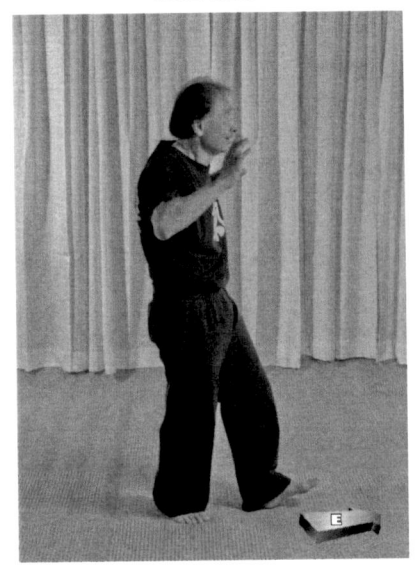

POSTURE 52-*INHALE*
Raise hands up in front, palms down, to shoulder height and then circle back towards chest, ending palms facing forward.

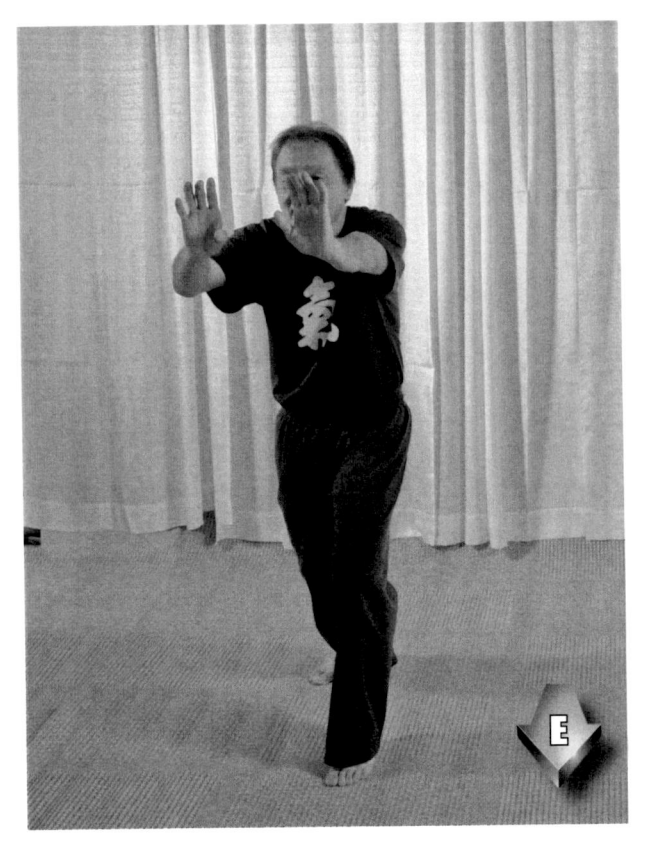

SIDE VIEW

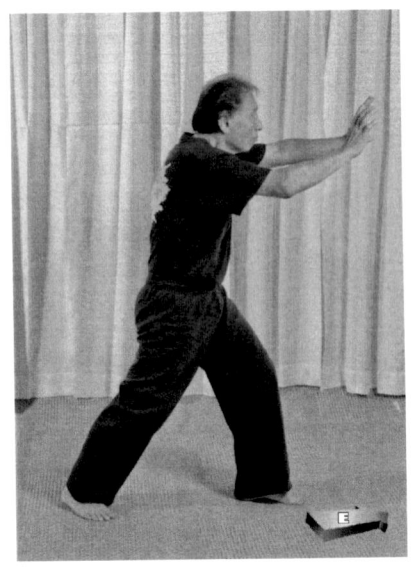

POSTURE 52-*EXHALE*
With palms facing forward, extend hands forward as LF steps into BS.

Posture 53

FRONT VIEW

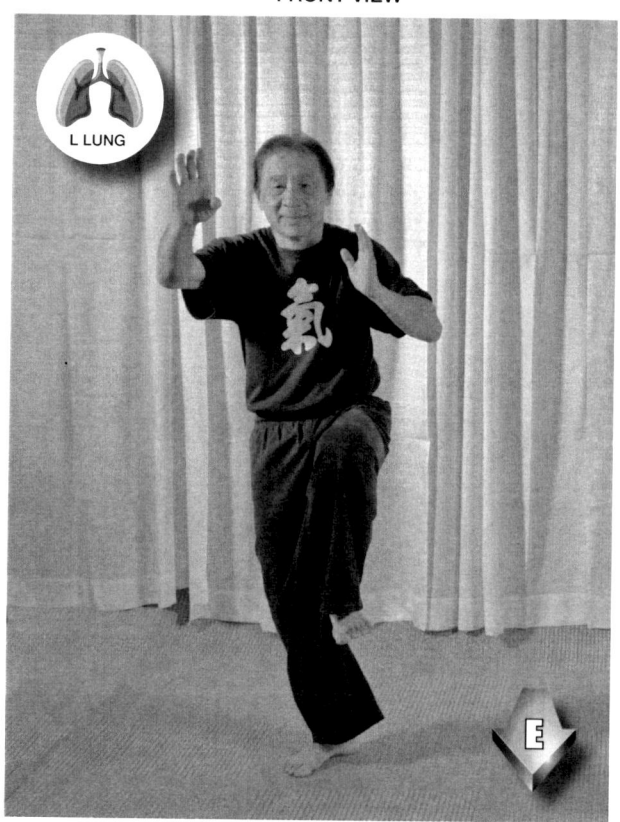

SIDE VIEW

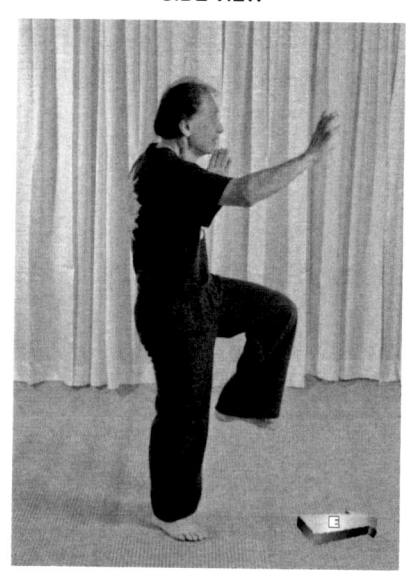

POSTURE 53-*INHALE*
LF raises as LH comes back to left shoulder, then body rotates to left. RH stays extended to front.

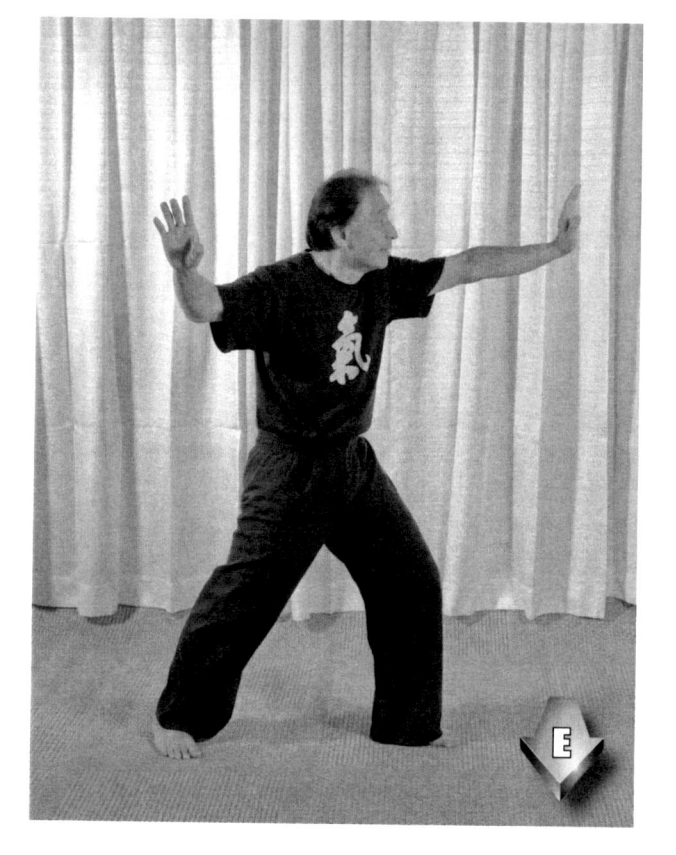

SIDE VIEW

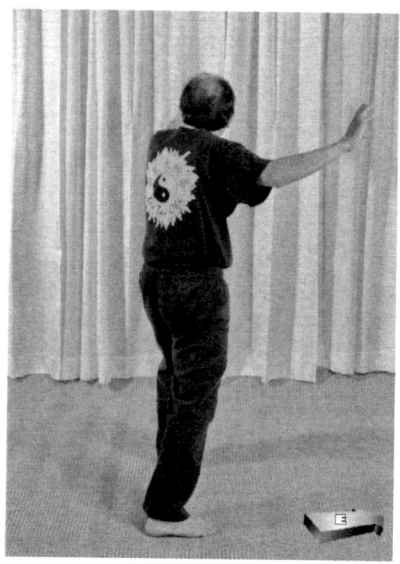

POSTURE 53-*EXHALE*
LF steps 90° to left and LH presses palm forward. RH stays in same position.

Posture 54

FRONT VIEW

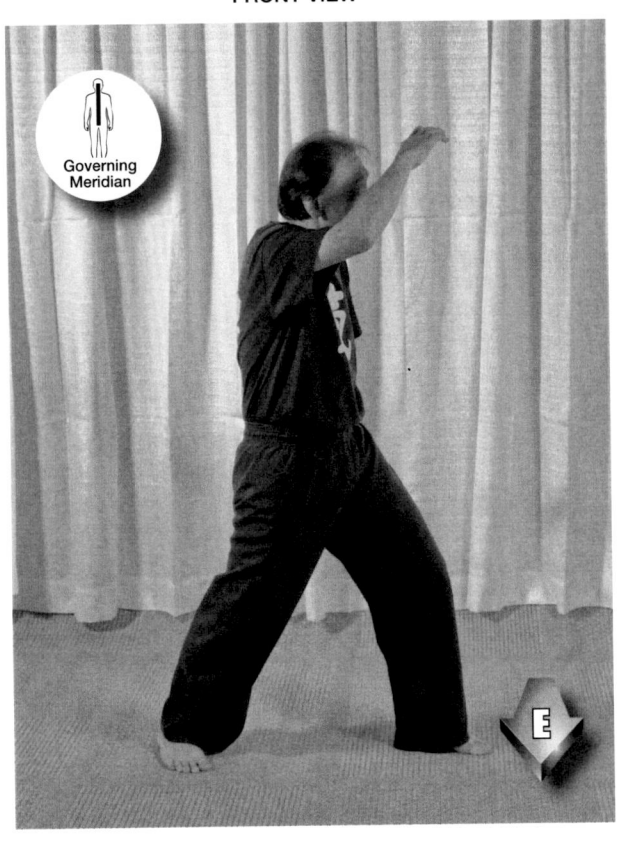

SIDE VIEW

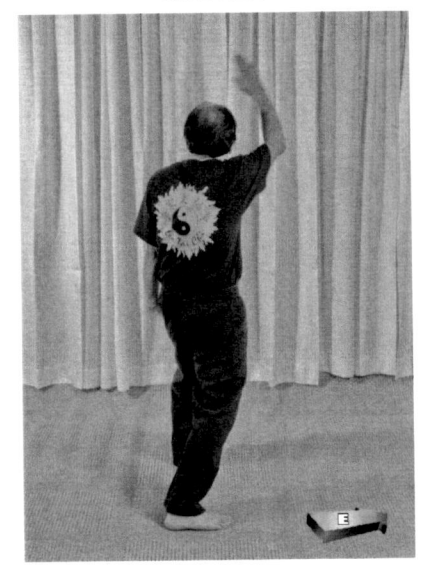

POSTURE 54-*INHALE*
RH crosses in front of body as LH circles out to the left side.

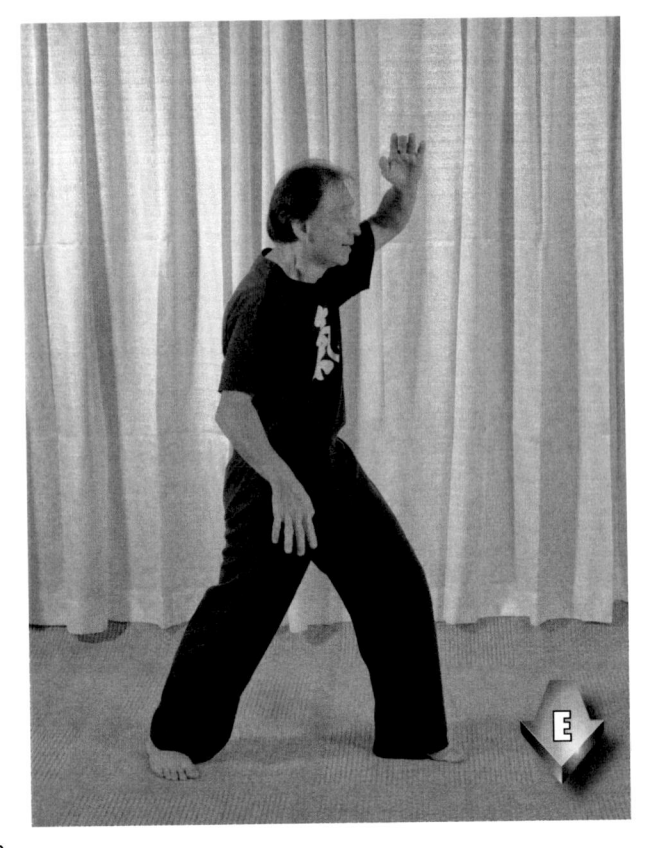

SIDE VIEW

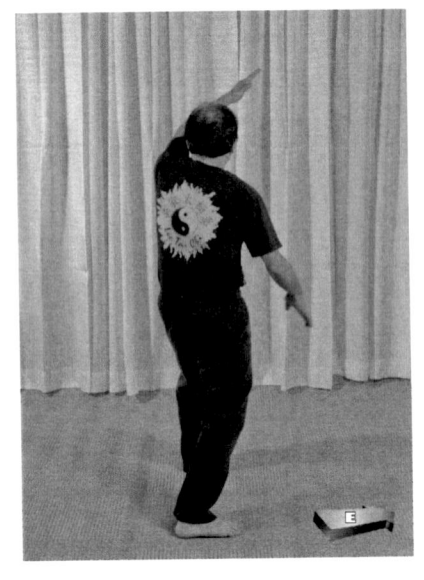

POSTURE 54-*EXHALE*
LH crosses in front of body as RH circles out to the right side.

Posture 55

FRONT VIEW

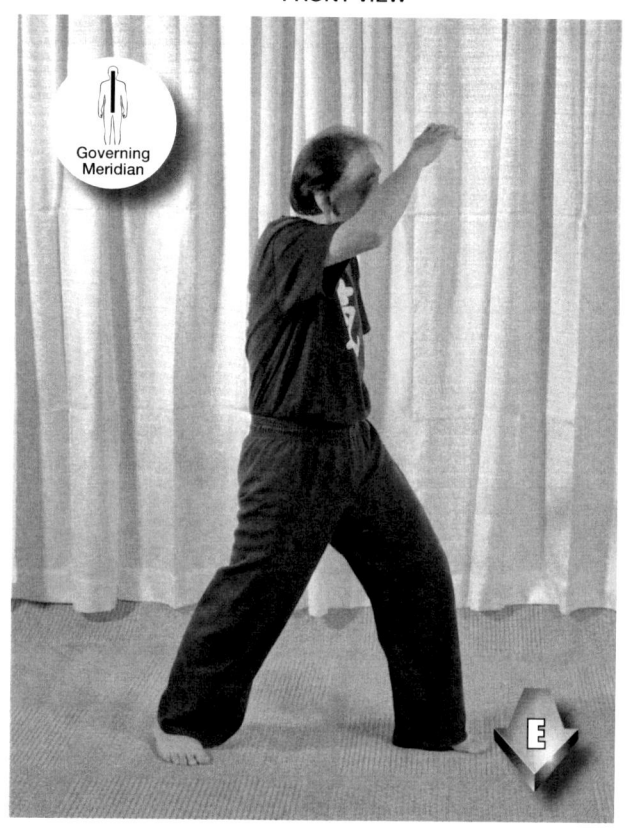

SIDE VIEW

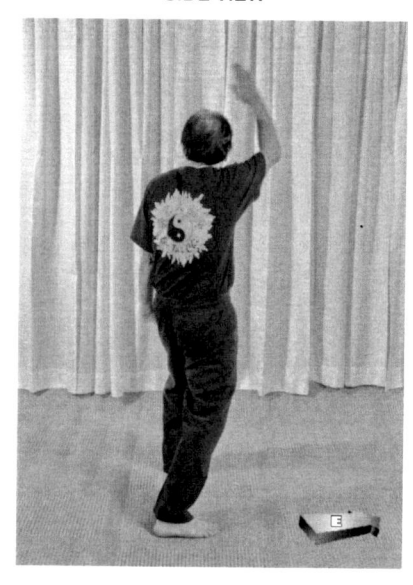

POSTURE 55-*INHALE*
RH crosses in front of body as LH circles out to the left side.

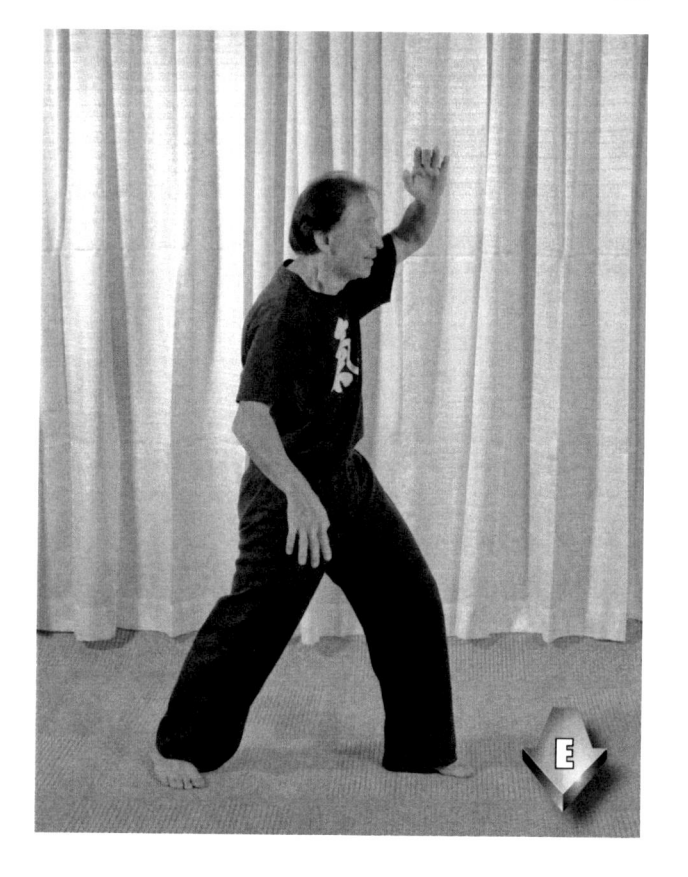

SIDE VIEW

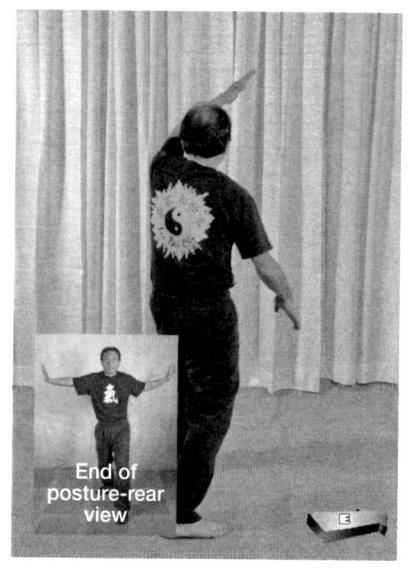

End of posture-rear view

POSTURE 55-*EXHALE*
LH crosses in front of body as RH circles out to the right side. End posture with both arms out to the side and fingers pointing up.

Posture 56

FRONT VIEW

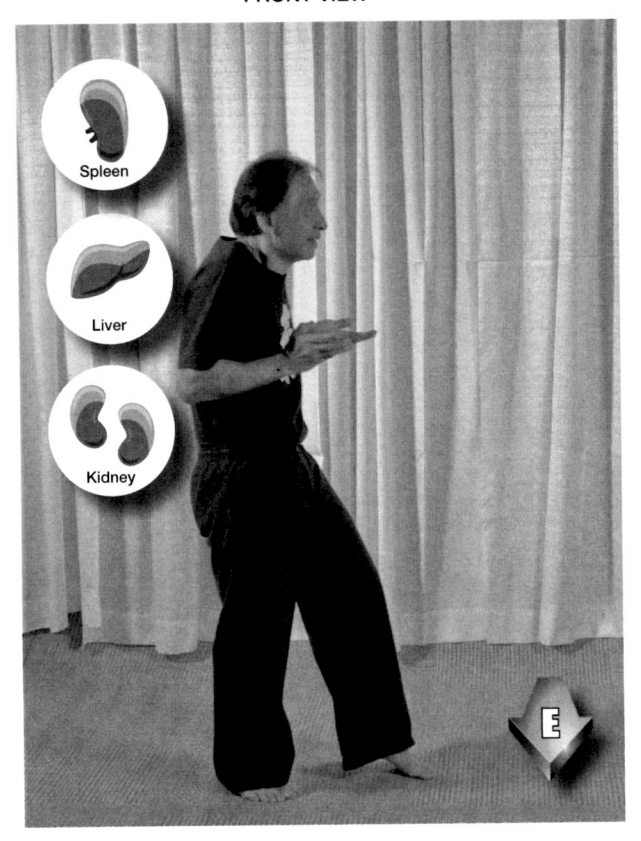

SIDE VIEW

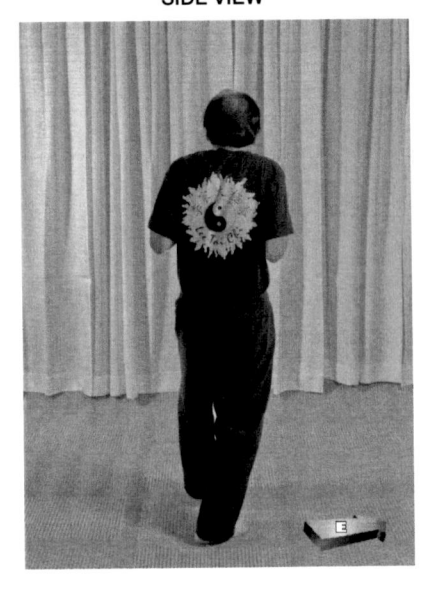

POSTURE 56-*INHALE*
Weight shifts to RF as both hands circle up and out to the side, as LF moves back to CS. Hands continue inward to chest level, palms up.

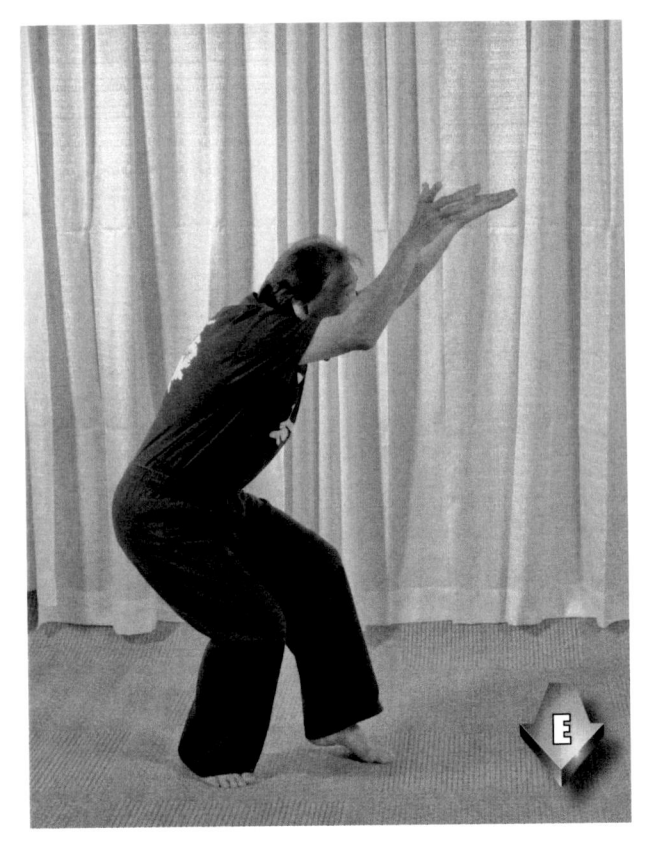

SIDE VIEW

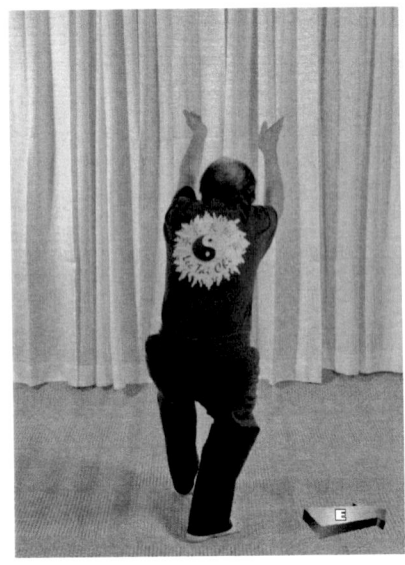

POSTURE 56-*EXHALE*
As you sink your stance, arms extend up above head with palms facing up.

Posture 57

FRONT VIEW

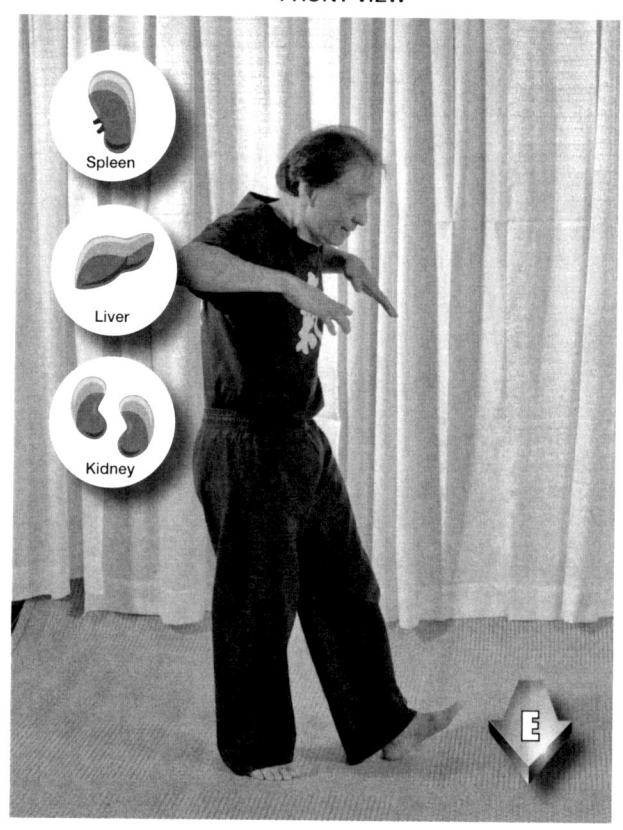

SIDE VIEW

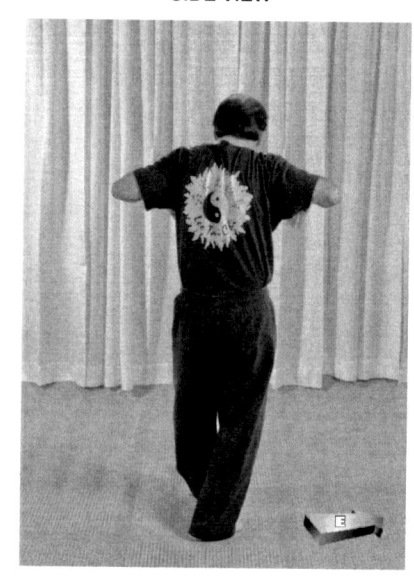

POSTURE 57-*INHALE*
LF moves to a heel stance as you rotate hands palms down and bring them in to the body, chest level.

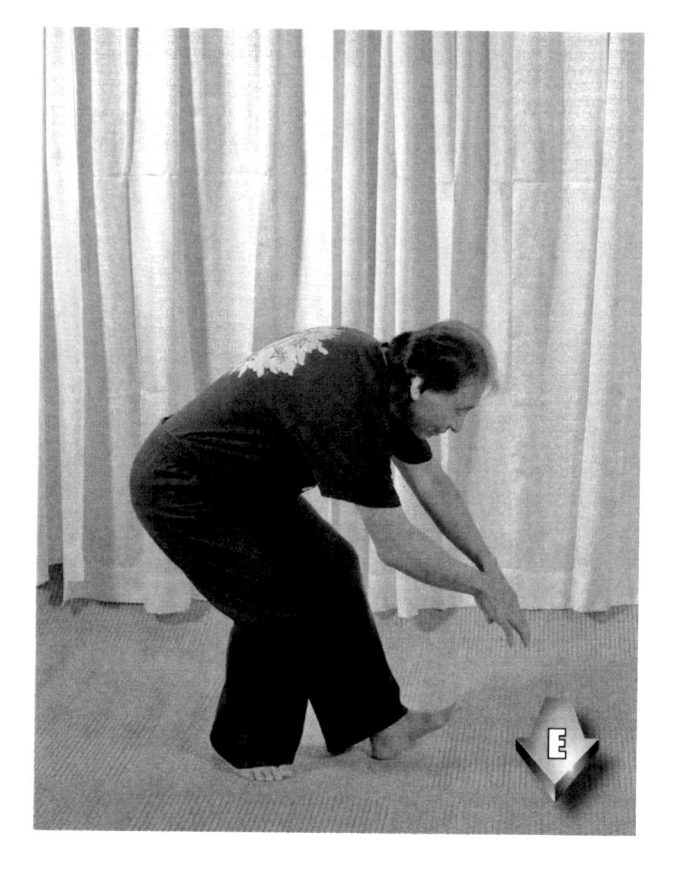

SIDE VIEW

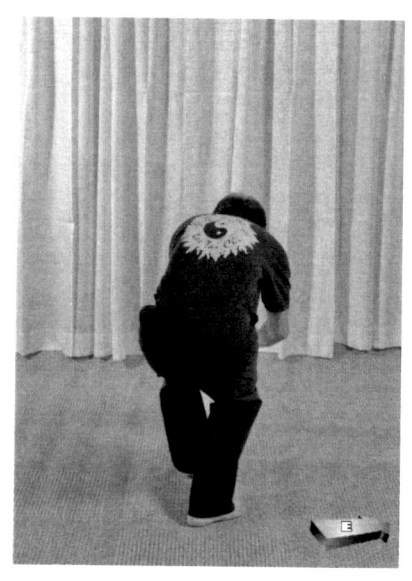

POSTURE 57-*EXHALE*
Hands extend down with fingertips 45° in front of the body as stance sinks.

Posture 58

FRONT VIEW

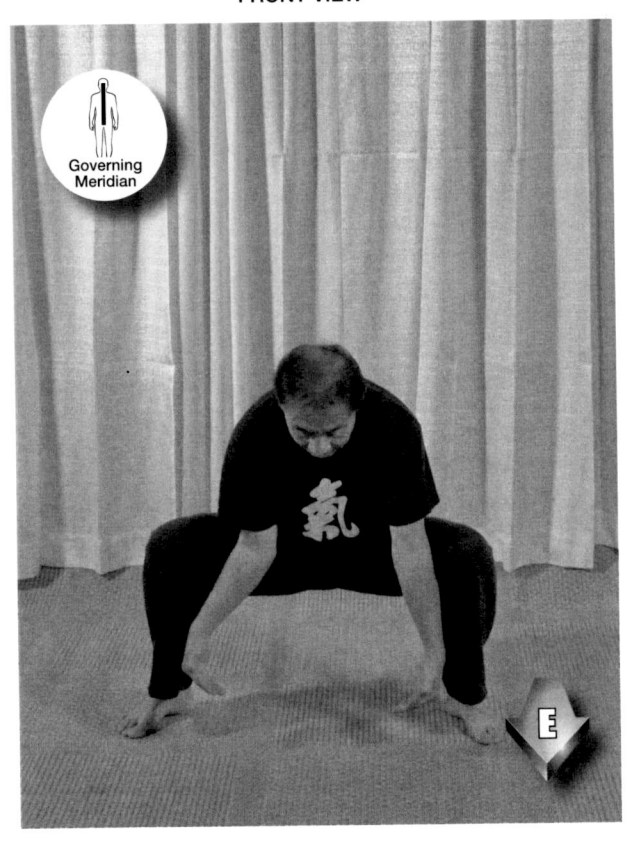

Governing Meridian

SIDE VIEW

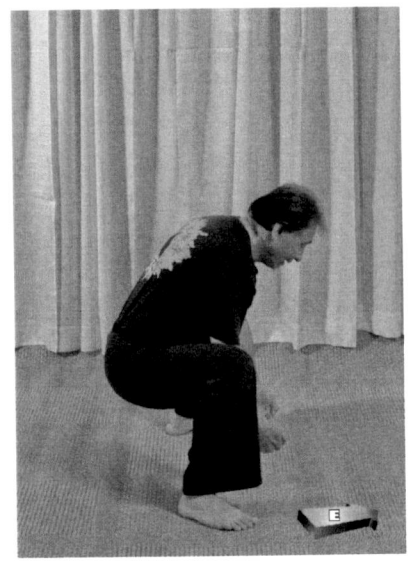

POSTURE 58-*INHALE*
LF steps to left into HS as hands reach out to the sides then in, palms up, as if grabbing a large box. (Knees are bent)

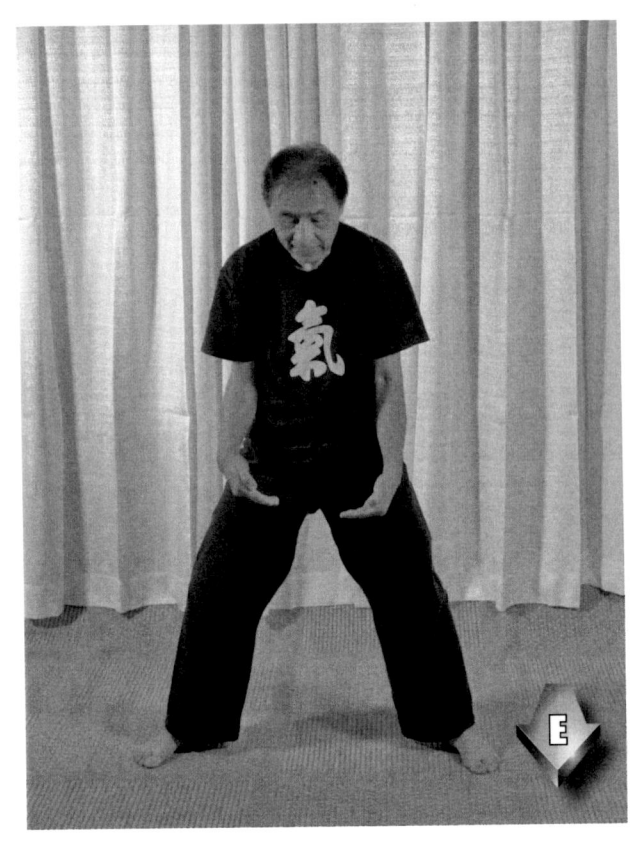

SIDE VIEW

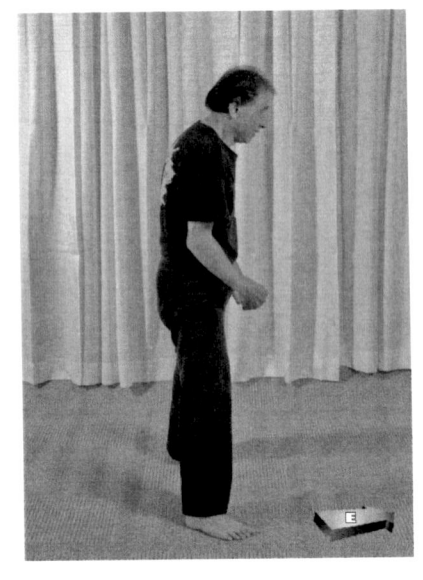

POSTURE 58-*EXHALE*
Raise stance as hands lift upwards to waist level.

Posture 59

FRONT VIEW

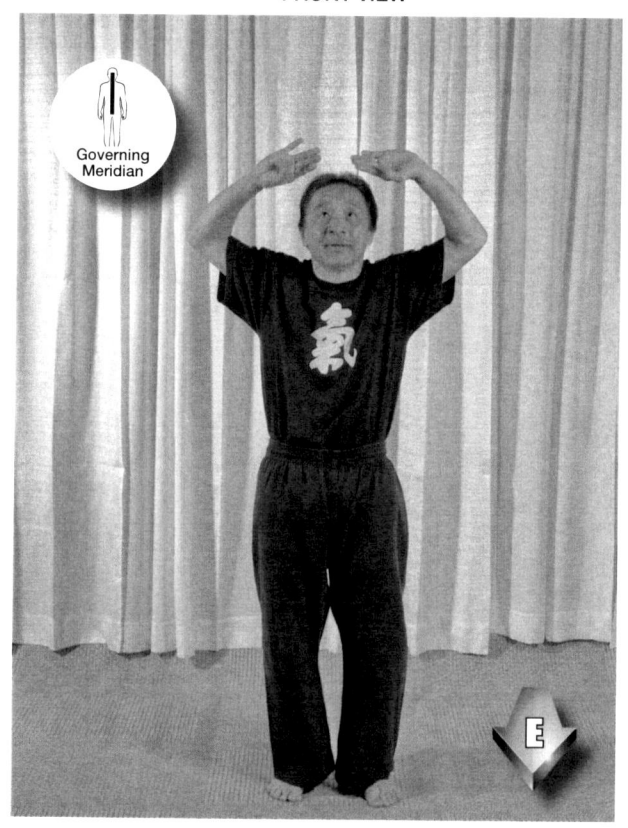

Governing Meridian

SIDE VIEW

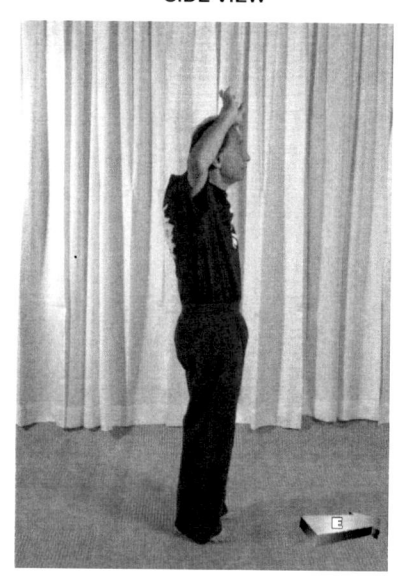

POSTURE 59-*INHALE*
RF steps in next to LF as body continues to rise hands come to shoulder level turning palms up.

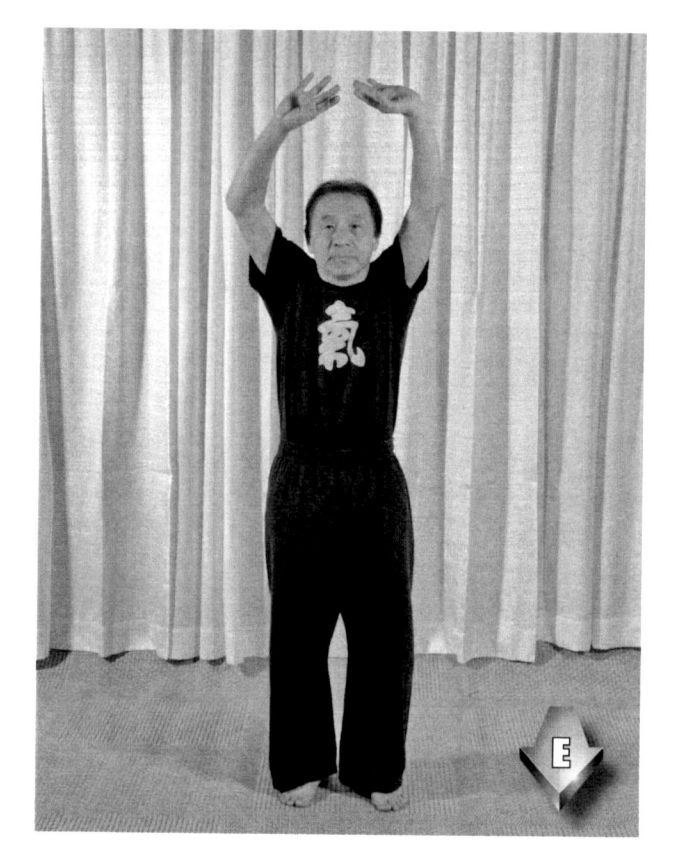

SIDE VIEW

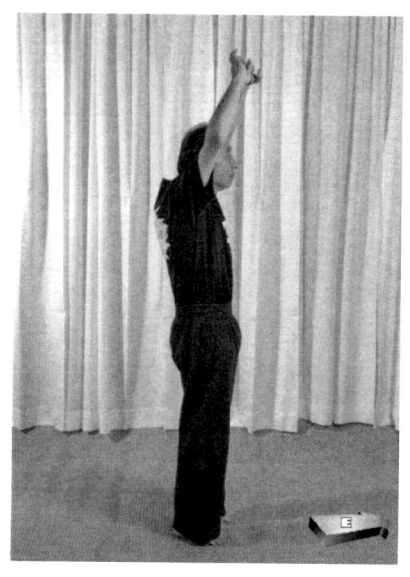

POSTURE 59-*EXHALE*
Hands extend up with palms facing up.

Posture 60

FRONT VIEW

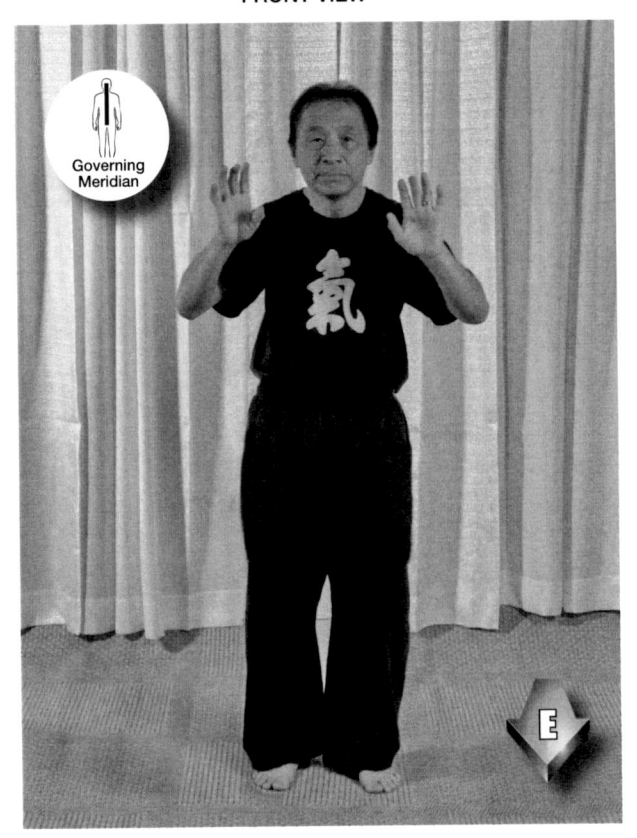

SIDE VIEW

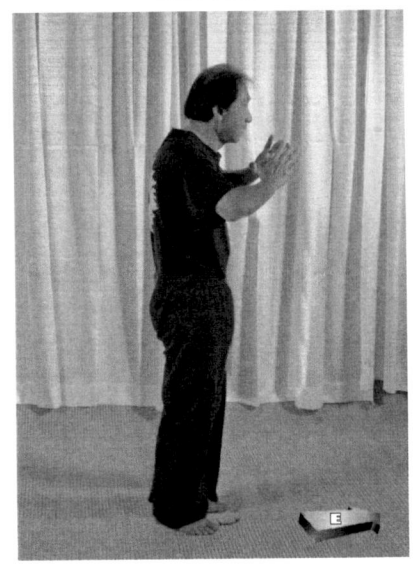

POSTURE 60-*INHALE*
Hands come down to shoulder level as palms turn to face forward.

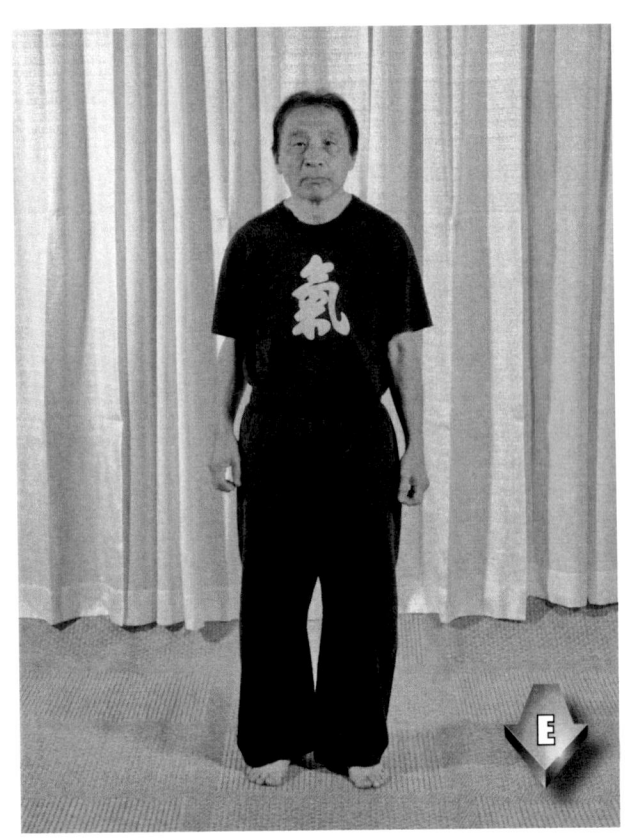

POSTURE 60-*EXHALE*
Hands continue to move down to the sides of the body as palms turn down, then come to rest down at the sides. Close with a bow.

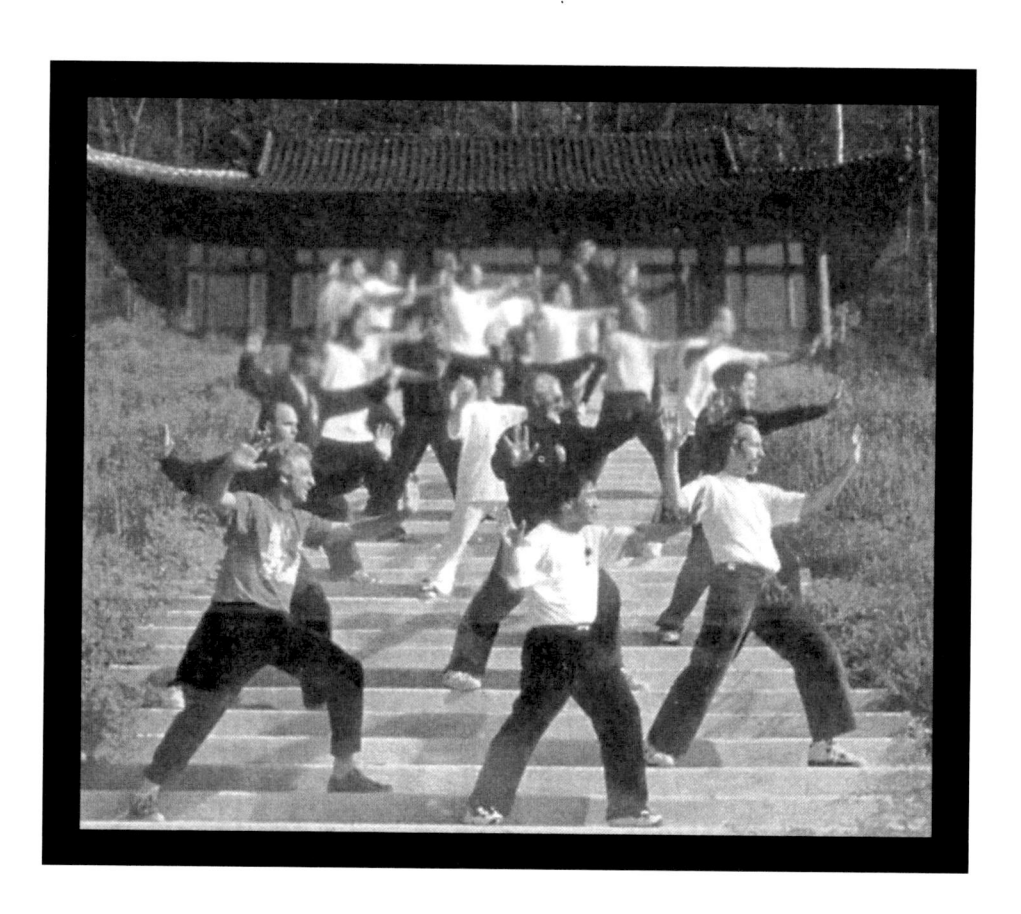

© Dean Hill Photography

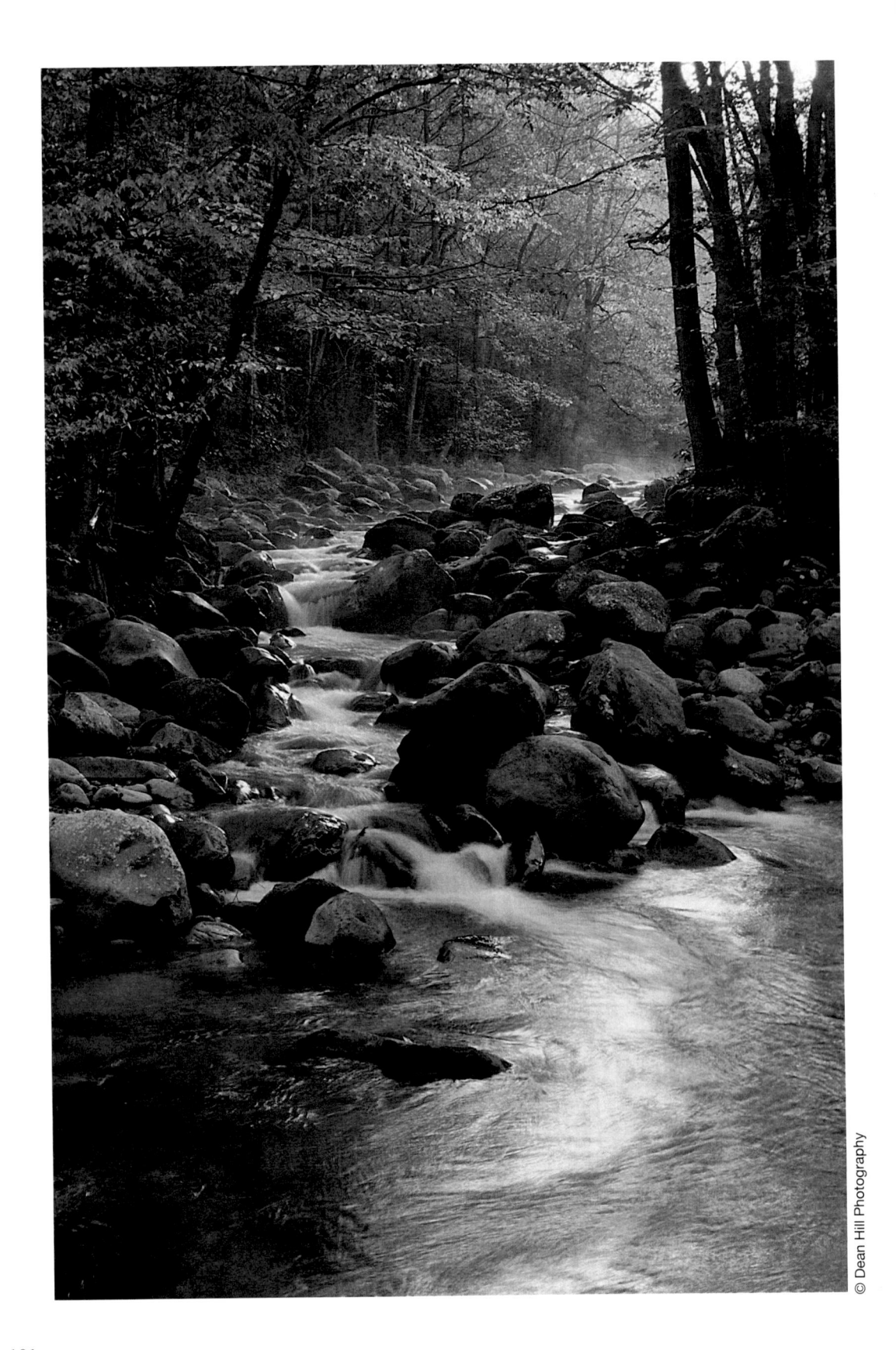

SIX

BREATHING

ONE OF THE MOST IMPORTANT PRINCIPLES OF TAI CHI PRACTICE IS YOUR BREATHING. Proper breathing while doing the form transforms Tai Chi from a relaxing, physical movement into a meditative powerhouse. The breath is the catalyst that helps generate your Chi, or life force, and provides the internal energy that is so important in attaining the benefits that Tai Chi practice offers.

Modern science says we can exist for close to 90 days without food, and perhaps 14 days without water. But how long can you last without breathing?

Fortunately, the breathing techniques are not complicated and can become almost second nature with time and repetition. Another benefit is that the same breathing techniques used for Tai Chi are also good for improving your everyday health. Just keep in mind to always listen to your body and let it tell you what is happening inside.

Inhale/Exhale

As you can see from the Tai Chi form description in the Forms chapter, each posture has an inhale and an exhale component. Each posture starts with the inhale portion, then finishes with the exhale portion. In Chinese Taoist philosophy, the inhale portion is referred to as the Yin side and the exhale portion as the Yang side (See the Yin-Yang section of the Philosophy chapter).

The timing on the inhale and exhale movements are identical, so if you are doing the inhale portion of the movement for, as an example, five seconds, you would perform the exhale portion of the posture for five seconds. If you are doing the inhale portion of the movement for six seconds, you would therefore perform the exhale portion of the posture for six seconds. It is important that this timing is maintained throughout the form, from beginning to end, helping to establish a rhythm, balance, and smooth pace.

I usually like to either count aloud if I am with a class or just count silently to myself while I am going through the form to help maintain a good, consistent pace.

-I will slowly count "1-2-3" as I do the inhale portion of the posture

-Then slowly count "1-2-3" as I do the exhale portion of the posture.

If each of the above "counts" is about two seconds long, then the entire inhale portion is six seconds total and the exhale portion is six seconds total. Keeping that up for the form's entire 60 postures would result in a duration of 12 minutes total, a good, average pace.

As you train more and gain more breathing capacity, you can increase the length of the inhale and exhale to extend the total time. It is usually good to keep the increase at about one count per inhale and one count per exhale for each posture as you advance. If the three count/six second pace is too challenging, you can reduce the pace to a two count/four second pace for each inhale and exhale.

And remember the most important part—breathe in, breathe out, and smile.

TIP: *Timing-* Imagine the rhythmic count of your breathing and heartbeat being akin to a drummer in a band. The steady pace of the breath — like a drummer's steady beat that provides the necessary cues to the rest of the band, so everyone plays together and not too fast or slow — helps unify body, mind and spirit so that the movements flow seamlessly.

In Through The Nose, Out Through The Mouth

When inhaling, breathe in through the nose. When exhaling, breathe out through the mouth. The nose provides an excellent filtering system to process the incoming breath and the oxygen-rich air stimulates the soft tissues of the upper respiratory system. **TIP:** The companion video's form section indicates the inhale and exhale portion of each posture with either a letter "I" or an "E" in the upper left hand corner of the screen.

A Start: Breathe Naturally

The best way to begin to add breathing to the Tai Chi form is to just breathe naturally. Use the above guidelines for which movements call for an inhale and which movements call for an exhale, including the balanced timing on the inhale and exhale portions. Especially when first learning the form, your attention is more likely on performing the physical movements correctly, so adding the awareness of inhaling and exhaling with the different postures is a great way to start.

Lower Level/Tan Tien Level Breathing

In addition to the timing of the breath, ***where*** you focus your breath is also important. There are two methods you can use to help focus your breath while practicing Tai Chi.

The first method is lower level or Tan Tien breathing. The term Tan Tien can be translated as "the Source Point" or "Main Field" being the main area of the body that can

Breathing

generate or store Chi. The Tan Tien is considered the source of human energy. Chinese Chi Kung practice uses three areas or levels in the body as points of focus, with the lower one located about one to two inches below your navel and three to four inches inward depending upon the individual. This lower level method is the best one to do once you are comfortable breathing naturally as described above. This next step of breathing with the Lower Level is a bit easier because your focus is just on a single area, but is no less an excellent method to generate powerful and effective internal strength.

-With this lower level method, start by imagining or visualizing the air traveling *downward* along a path from your nose to the lower Tan Tien, about one to two inches below your navel on the inhale portion. As you inhale, slowly count to yourself "1-2-3."

-Then imagine or visualize the air traveling *upward* along the same path on the exhale portion. As you exhale, slowly count to yourself "1-2-3."

Inhale

-With practice, you try to feel the lower level expanding with the inhale and upon arrival of the air, then the lower level contracting with the exhale as the air leaves and your attention moves upward with the exiting air.

-The breath should be smooth and continue throughout the entire inhale or exhale portion with no change of speed.

The volume of air should come as close to being 100 percent full on the inhale portion and 100 percent empty on the exhale, but *without any strain or tension.* If you feel

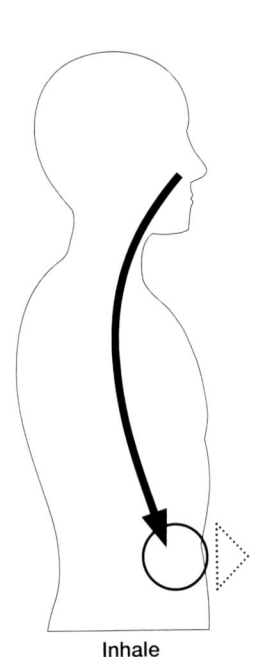

Exhale

yourself tensing in order to feel full or empty, it is better to reduce the volume. A good practice when just starting Tai Chi training is to aim for about 80 percent full or empty at the beginning, then gradually work up to 90 percent, then to completely full or empty over time as you feel more relaxed and comfortable with the greater volume.

The Natural Complete Breath

Another breathing method is called the Natural Complete Breath, utilizing all three levels: lower, center, and upper. The center level is located near the solar plexus, and the upper level is located in the upper lung/chest area.

-Like the lower level breathing technique described above, you imagine or visualize the air traveling down along a path from your nose to the lower level on the initial portion of the inhale

-Then, while continuing the inhale, move to the center level, and finish the inhale with focus on the upper level.

-At each level, expand that spot as the air fills that specific level. As an example, on a six-count paced inhale/exhale you would focus on

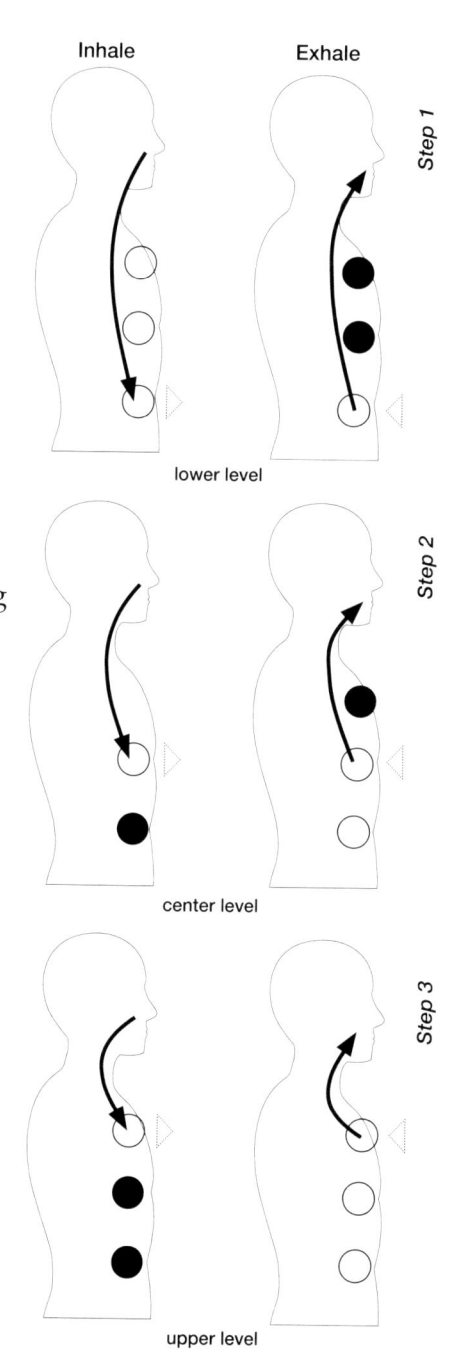

Breathing

the lower level for count one-two, the center level for count three-four, and the upper level for count five-six. As you move from one level to the other, you maintain the volume of air in each previous level.

On the exhale, the order of focus is the same. Start at the lower level exhaling for the one-two count, visualizing the air traveling *upward*, then the center level for three-four count, then finishing the exhale at the upper level on the five-six count. At each level, contract that spot as the air leaves that area of the body and keep that level empty.

> **DID YOU KNOW?**
>
> **Imagine your lungs as a water bottle in the Complete Breath.**
>
> To help visualize the Complete Breath, imagine your lungs as a bottle of water. When filling the bottle with water (air), the bottom of the bottle fills first, followed by the center, then the top of the bottle. When you tip the bottle over to empty, it empties from the bottom first, then the center, and finally the top.

Developing Effective Breathing

One of the best ways to develop your breathing skills for Tai Chi is to do separate breathing exercises outside of the form's practice. We like to use a number of training exercises that are a part of a larger field of study called Chi Kung, translated as "energy work."

PACE & VOLUME OF AIR: For all of the following exercises, decide on a comfortable pace that you can maintain without straining or becoming lightheaded. A three count inhale and a three count exhale is often a good pace, with each single count being about two seconds long for a total of six seconds inhaling and six seconds exhaling. If counting "1-2-3" for six seconds is too much, reduce to a three count that is about five seconds long or even more to a two count (four seconds) on the inhale and a two count on the exhale, then practice until your capacity grows over time.

TIP: Set the timer on your phone for comfortable duration while doing the following exercises. This allows you to clear your mind of the thought of how long you've been practicing or how much more time you have to go, which can be very distracting. Start with a two or three minute duration for each exercise, then gradually increase by one minute each week. Always be 100 percent alert when doing these exercises.

EXERCISE ONE: Lower Level Breathing (Standing or Sitting) *See illustration in Lower Level/Tan Tien Breathing section on page 105.*

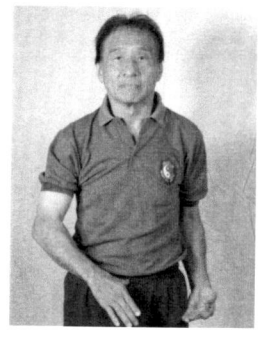

Lower Level

-Start in a relaxed standing or sitting position. The back should be naturally straight and head raised, but keep the body from becoming tense.

-Place the palm of one hand on the lower level/Tan Tien, about one to two inches below your navel. (You can omit this part by removing the hand once you feel comfortable isolating the lower level.)

-Close the eyes and take a long cleansing inhale and exhale.

-Then inhale through the nose and visualize the air traveling down along a path from your nose to the lower level/Tan Tien where your hand is located.

-As you inhale, slowly count to yourself "1-2-3" as you visualize the air moving downward.

-Feel the lower level expanding with the inhale and upon

arrival of the air.

-Once full at the count of three, then slowly start to exhale at the same rate as you inhaled.

-As you exhale, slowly count to yourself "1-2-3" as you visualize the air moving upward.

-Contract the lower level as you feel the air exiting and moving upward.

Repeat

EXERCISE TWO: Complete Breath-Upper Level Only (Standing or Sitting)

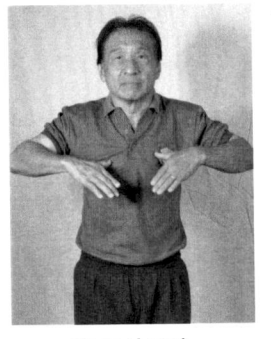

Upper Level

When starting to train for the Complete Breath, begin by working on just one level at a time. We already isolated the lower level in the first exercise. This time, just focus on the upper level, in the chest. This is often the easiest level to begin with as it is how most people breathe without training.

-Start in a relaxed standing or sitting position. The back should be naturally straight and head raised, but keep the body from becoming tense.

-Close the eyes and take a long cleansing inhale and exhale.

-Place the thumbs of both hands on the upper level, chest area. (You can omit this part by removing the hand once you feel comfortable isolating the Upper level.)

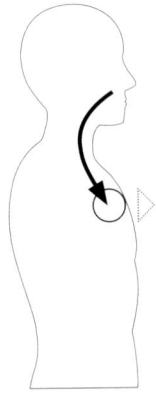

Inhale

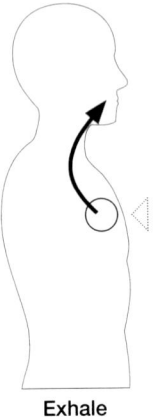

Exhale

-Then inhale through the nose and visualize the air traveling down along a path from your nose to the upper level, chest area where your thumbs are located.

-As you inhale, slowly count to yourself "1-2-3" as you visualize the air moving downward.

-Feel the upper level expand with the inhale and upon arrival of the air.

-Once full at the count of three, then slowly start to exhale at the same rate as you inhaled.

-As you exhale, slowly count to yourself "1-2-3" as you visualize the air moving upward.

-Contract the upper level as you feel the air exiting and moving upward.

Repeat

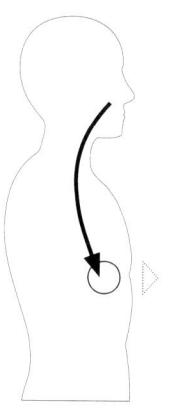

EXERCISE THREE: Complete Breath-Center Level Only (Standing or Sitting)

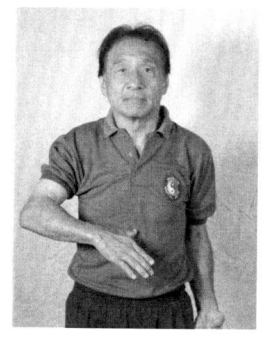

Center Level

-Start in a relaxed standing or sitting position. The back should be naturally straight and head raised, but keep the body from becoming tense.

-Close the eyes and take a long cleansing inhale and exhale.

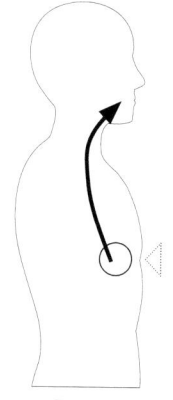

Inhale

Exhale

-Place the thumb of one hand on the center level around your solar plexus. (You can omit this part by removing the hand once you feel comfortable isolating the center level.)

Breathing

-Then inhale through the nose and visualize the air traveling down along a path from your nose to the center level.

-As you inhale, slowly count to yourself "1-2-3" as you visualize the air moving downward.

-Feel the center level expand with the inhale and upon the arrival of the air.

-Once full, then slowly exhale at the same rate as you inhaled, with the focus starting at the center level.

-As you exhale, slowly count to yourself "1-2-3" as you visualize the air moving upward.

-Contract the center level as you feel the air exiting and moving upward.

-Repeat

EXERCISE FOUR: Complete Breath-All Three Levels (Standing or Sitting) *See illustration in* The Natural Complete Breath *section on page 106.)*

-Start in a relaxed standing or sitting position. The back should be naturally straight and head raised, but keep the body from becoming tense.

-Close the eyes and take a long cleansing inhale and exhale.

-Then inhale through the nose and visualize the air traveling down along a path from your nose to the lower level, about one to two inches below your navel.

-As you inhale, slowly count to yourself "1-2-3" as you visualize the air moving downward.

-On the "one" feel the lower level expanding with the inhale and arrival of the air.

-As you count two, feel the air move up to the center level, expanding at the solar plexus.

-As you count three, feel the air move up to the upper level, expanding at the chest.

-Once full, slowly exhale at the same rate as you inhaled, with the focus starting at the lower level.

-As you exhale, slowly count to yourself "1-2-3" as you visualize the air moving upward.

-On the "one," feel the lower level contracting with the exhale as the air leaves the lower level.

-As you count two, feel the exiting air move up to the center level, contracting at the solar plexus.

-As you count three, feel the exiting air move up to the upper level, contracting at the chest.

-Repeat, inhaling to the lower level to start the sequence.

Because the all-level, Complete Breath is a bit more complex for beginners, practicing these Chi Kung exercises outside of the form practice is an excellent way to develop your breathing skills before applying the Complete Breath method to Tai Chi.

HOW TO IMPROVE: Once you can comfortably perform a three count for the above exercises, add one more "beat," inhaling/exhaling for a four count to increase your capacity. Practice until this volume becomes comfortable, then increase the timing to a five count, and so-on. Make sure, though, not to add any physical tension when attempting to increase the length of the breath.

Breathing

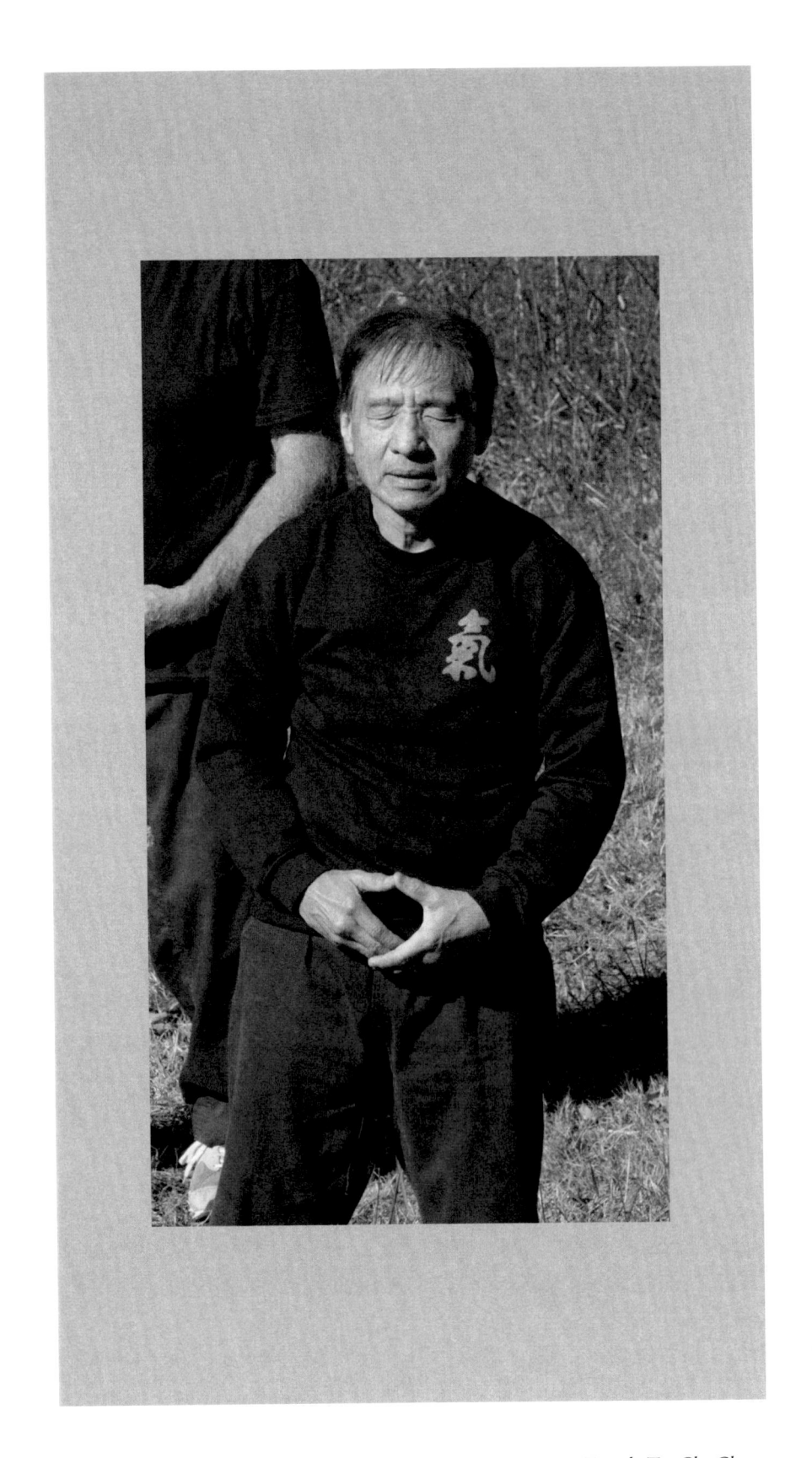

Lee Family Tai Chi Chuan

PAO SHEN TA CH'IAO

Making a Connection Within Yourself

An important basic meditative position, whether for Lee Family Tai Chi training or for general meditation practice, is called *Pao Shen Ta Ch'iao*. Pao Shen is translated as "To Protect Life" and Ta Ch'iao is translated as "The Great Bridge." Together, they mean "The Great Connection." "Protect Life" comes from the main area of focus and location of the hands during the posture that is near the navel where the umbilical cord was attached to our mothers in the womb. This is where we received our oxygen and nourishment that sustained us until we entered the outside world. This is also where the Tan Tien is located, the main source of our Chi. Ta Ch'iao or "Great Bridge" refers to the position of the tip of tongue touching the roof of the mouth just behind the upper teeth with the tip pointing up towards the nose, creating a connection or bridge between the upper and lower body.

Pao Shen Ta Ch'iao is an excellent method to mediate in a simple, but effective way either before or after doing the Tai Chi form, or any other time when a calm and peaceful state is desired. The main goal of Pao Shen Ta Ch'iao meditation is to make a good connection within yourself. We want to clear the mind and move our awareness inward, sensing our breath, our heartbeat, and releasing any tension.

The Pao Shen Ta Ch'iao position can be done either standing, sitting, or laying down. In this position, the back of the right hand is placed so that it rests in the palm of the left hand. The tips of the two thumbs are then connected, forming a small circular opening just below the thumbs. When standing, the hands are positioned with the right palm resting against the body and the center of the circular shape rests over the Tan Tien area, one to two inches below the naval. When sitting, rest the hands comfortably in the lap, palms up, and the back of the left hand touching the body. Place the tip of the tongue to the roof of the mouth just behind the upper front teeth with the tip of the tongue pointing up.

This breathing pattern is much like the Lower Level Tan Tien Breathing covered on page 104, *but is done more lightly with an emphasis on releasing any physical tension, especially on the exhale portion of the breath.* Listen to or feel your heartbeat to set the pace of your breathing. *Be as peaceful as you can.* This type of lower level breathing is also more natural, much like a newborn baby's breathing.

EXERCISE: Pao Shen Ta Ch'iao Breathing (Standing or Sitting)

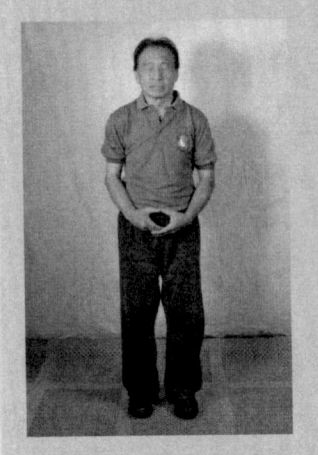

-Start in a relaxed standing or sitting position. The back should be straight and head raised, but keep the body from becoming tense. Place the hands as described above.

-Close the eyes and take a long cleansing inhale and exhale.

-Keep a light focus within the mind, behind your eyes, throughout the exercise, creating an empty, calm space. This is targeting the hippocampus area of the brain.

-Then inhale through the nose and visualize the air traveling down along a path from your nose to the Tan Tien, about one to two inches below your navel.

-As you inhale, slowly count to yourself "1-2-3" as you visualize the air moving downward. This is about a six second pace.

-Once you complete the count of three, slowly start to exhale at the same rate as you inhaled.

-As you exhale, slowly count to yourself "1-2-3" as you visualize the air moving upward. Relax the body on the exhale, with an emphasis on any tension or stress exiting your body.

-Repeat

After spending some time training with this exercise, you will be able to create an almost automatic, unconscious state of breathing and inner calmness in this position. One of the goals of all meditation is to put you in the here and now with your full awareness on what exists in the moment. In this meditative exercise, we want to achieve a state where we are just "being," without an inner dialogue or outer distractions, making that strong inner connection.

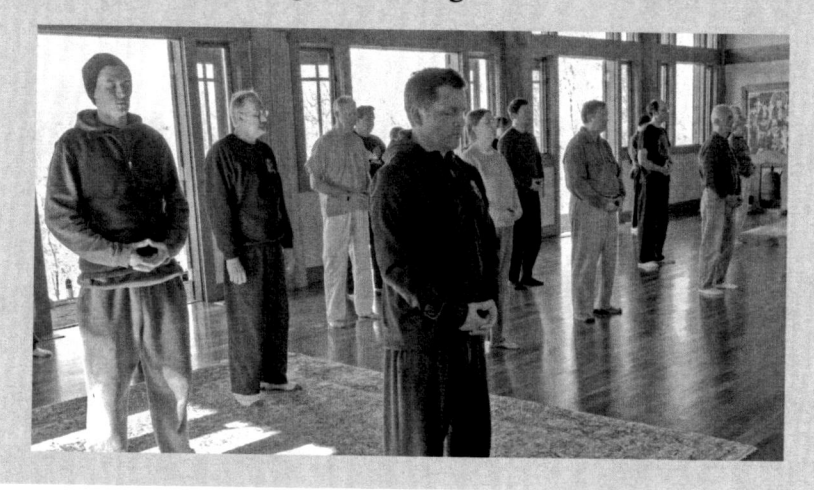

Breathing Exercises With Movement And Stances

The previous breathing exercises can be done either while standing or sitting, and are done without any external body movement. The following Chi Kung exercises use similar breathing techniques from those exercises, but are done with some simple physical motion and the body positioned in one of the stances used in Tai Chi. These exercises can help you to better coordinate your breath with your physical movement, improve seamlessness between postures, and develop a smoother, more fluid overall motion.

As with the previous exercises, decide on a comfortable pace that you can maintain without straining or becoming lightheaded. A three count inhale/exhale pace is a good starting point. For these exercises with motion, use the lower level breathing technique to start.

OPENING/CLOSING ROUTINE

This Opening/Closing routine combines the first and last postures of the Tai Chi form.

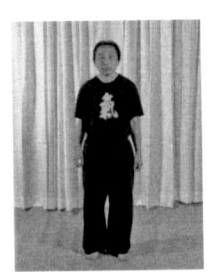

Start Inhale

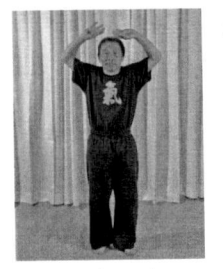

Inhale-end

Start in a standing position, feet placed about shoulder width apart, and your weight equally distributed 50/50 on both legs. Place your arms at your side with your palms facing your body.

1) As you inhale, move your arms out to the sides and up over your head until the fingertips point towards each other about six inches above your head. End with both palms facing upward. As in the previous exercises, inhale through the nose and visualize the air traveling down along a path from your nose to the lower level/Tan Tien, about one to two inches below your navel.

Exhale-end

2) As you exhale, extend both hands upward, palms facing toward the ceiling until your arms are straight (but do not lock the elbows). As in the previous exercises, exhale through the mouth as you visualize the air moving upward from the Tan Tien.

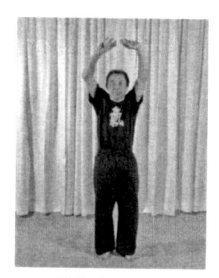

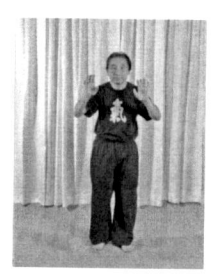

Inhale-end

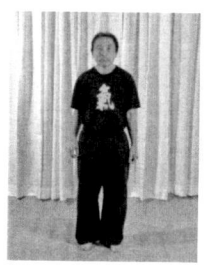

3) As you inhale, rotate your hands so that your palms are facing forward with fingers pointing up and slowly move your arms down to shoulder level. Inhale through the nose and visualize the air traveling down along a path from your nose to the Tan Tien.

Exhale-end

4) As you exhale, continue to move your hands down to the side of the body, turning the palms to face the body as in the starting position. Exhale through the mouth as you visualize the air moving upward from the Tan Tien.

Repeat

BO STANCE ROUTINE

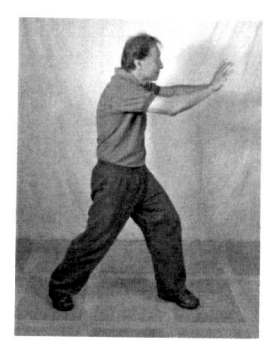

Bo Stance Routine- Start

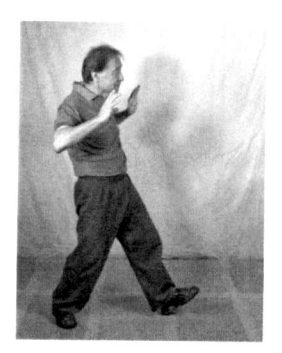

Bo Stance Routine- Inhale

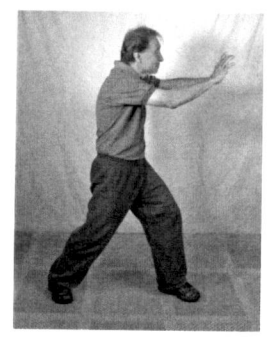

Bo Stance Routine- Exhale

From the Bo Stance position (see Stances Chapter) start with both arms extended to the front with palms facing forward.

Breathing

1) As you inhale, slowly shift your weight from the front leg to the rear leg, moving your arms/hands toward your body at chest level. The back remains vertical and the head is raised throughout the motion. Inhale and visualize the air traveling down along a path from your nose to the Tan Tien, about one to two inches below your navel.

2) As you exhale, slowly shift your weight from the rear leg back to the front leg, moving your arms/hands away your body, palms forward, until they reach just above the front foot. Exhale as you visualize the air moving upward from the Tan Tien.

Repeat

For the beginner, perform six full repetitions with the left leg forward and then six with the right leg forward. You can increase the number of repetitions as you practice over time. You can also slow the movement and increase the count/pace as you become more comfortable with the three count, adding one more "beat," inhaling/exhaling for a four count to increase your breathing capacity. Practice until this volume becomes comfortable, then increase the timing to a five count, and so-on. The greater the length of the breath, the more efficiently the system works.

HORSE STANCE ROUTINE

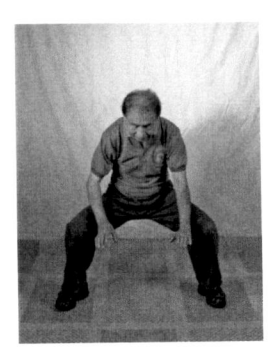

Horse Stance Routine- Start

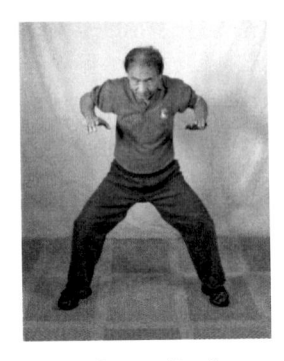

Horse Stance Routine- Inhale

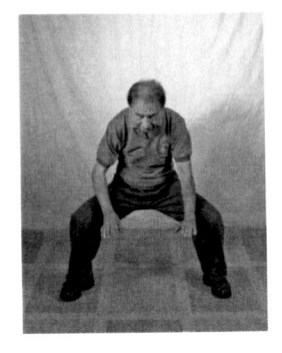

Horse Stance Routine- Exhale

From the Horse Stance position (see Stances Chapter) start with both arms extend downward just inside the thighs with palms facing toward the floor.

1) As you inhale, slowly raise your body, moving your arms/hands upward to chest level. The back remains vertical and the head is raised throughout the motion.

2) As you exhale, slowly bend the knees, lowering your stance while moving the hands downward with palms toward the floor, to reach the original starting position.

Repeat

For the beginner, perform six repetitions. You can increase the number of repetitions or slow the movement/increase the air volume as you practice over time.

CAT STANCE ROUTINE

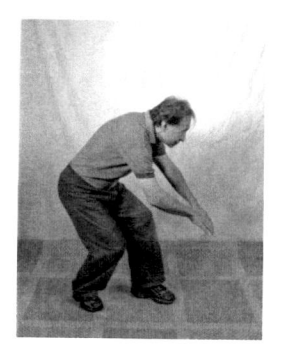

Cat Stance Routine- Start

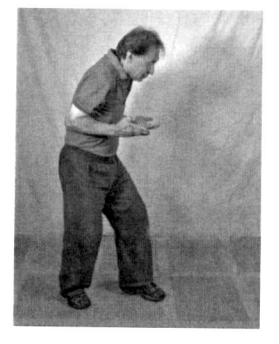

Cat Stance Routine- Inhale

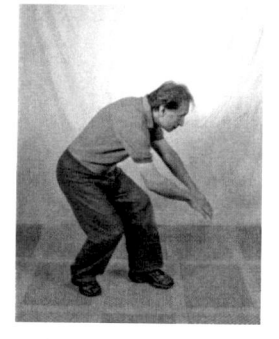

Cat Stance Routine- Exhale

From the Cat Stance position (see Stances Chapter) start with both arms extended downward around knee level, palms facing the body and fingers pointing down.

1) As you inhale, slowly raise your body, moving your arms/hands upward to waist level.

2) As you exhale, slowly bend the knees, lowering your stance while moving the hands downward, leading with the fingertips, to reach the original starting position.

Breathing

When deepening the stance, do not bend too much at the waist, keeping the lower back straight and the head raised throughout the motion.

Repeat

For the beginner, perform six repetitions with the left leg forward, then six with the right leg forward. You can increase the number of repetitions or slow the movement/increase the volume as you practice over time.

HEEL STANCE ROUTINE

Same as the Cat Stance routine, but the front foot contacts the floor with the heel rather than the ball of the foot.

BO/CAT STANCE ROUTINE

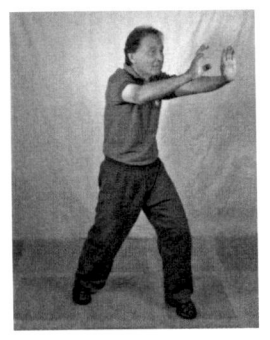

Bo/Cat Stance Routine- Start

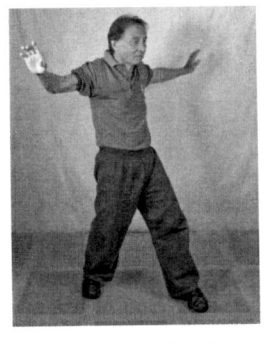

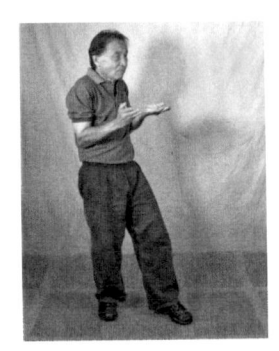

Bo/Cat Stance Routine- Inhale-1

Bo/Cat Stance Routine- Inhale-2

From the Bo Stance position (see Stances Chapter) start with both arms extended to the front, palms facing to the front.

1) As you inhale, shift your weight to the rear leg and circle the hands up, then back toward the outside of the body. Finish your inhale by bringing the hands inward in front of the chest with the palms facing up.

2) As you exhale, sink your stance by bending the knees and extending the hands up, palms facing up, above the head.

Bo/Cat Stance Routine- Exhale

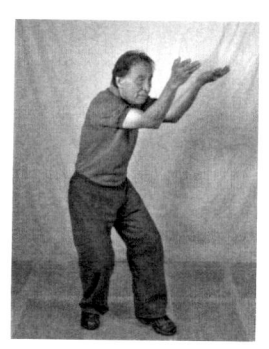

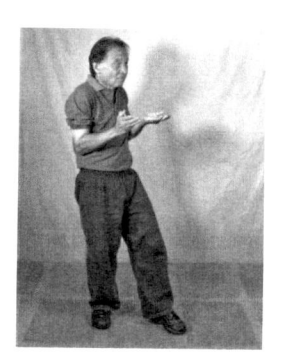

Bo/Cat Stance Routine- Inhale

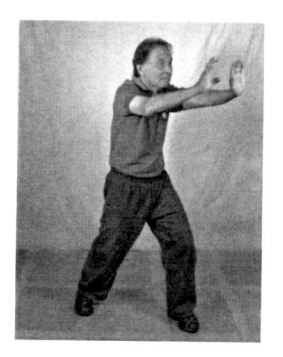

Bo/Cat Stance Routine- Exhale close

3) Inhale as you raise your stance and bring the hands back in front of the chest with the palms facing up.

4) Exhale as you step forward into a bo stance, with both arms extended to the front, palms facing to the front.

Repeat

For the beginner, perform six repetitions with the left leg forward, then six with the right leg forward. You can increase the number of repetitions or slow the movement/increase the volume as you practice over time.

Breathing

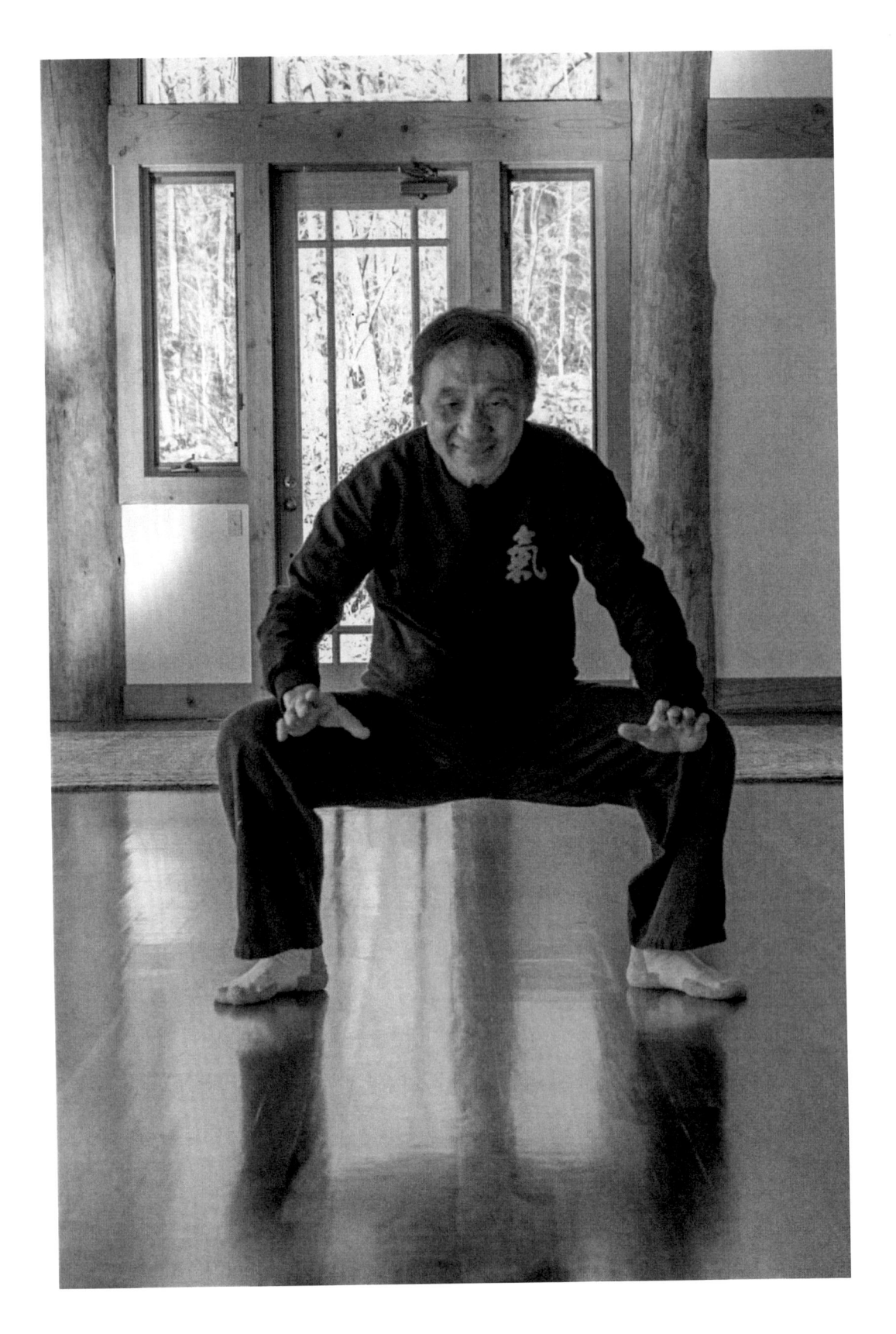

SEVEN

STANCES

THE STANCES USED IN LEE FAMILY TAI CHI establish an important foundation for the practice. Stability, balance, body alignment, and lower body strength—our entire body's equilibrium—are all improved from proper implementation and awareness of the body's position in these stances.

We utilize four main stances—the bo, horse, cat, and heel stance.

Bo Stance

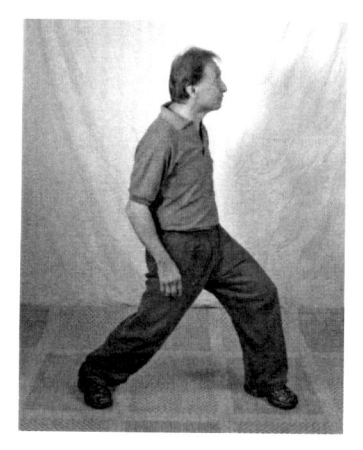

In the bo stance position, the front knee is bent, the rear leg is straight (but not locked), and the back is upright, similar to a lunge. The hips and shoulders face squarely forward. The distribution of weight is approximately 60 percent on the front leg and 40 percent on the rear leg. The bottoms of both feet are flat to the floor, with the toes of the rear foot pointing 60 degrees to the side opposite of the front leg, and the front foot's toes pointing 45 degrees to the side opposite of the front leg. The bo stance can be done with either the right or left leg as a front leg.

The amount of bend angle in the front leg can vary depending on the level of experience, strength, or physical limitations of the practitioner, but an angle of 45 to 80 degrees is recommended depending on the posture. Generally, the lower the better for the greatest stability and strength training, but deepening the stance to a full 90 degrees is not necessary for Tai Chi practice.

In the bo stance, the body's position is strongest from the front or rear, but not from the side.

Horse Stance

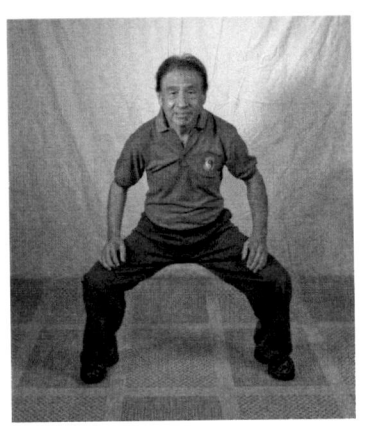

In the horse stance position, the feet are parallel with each other, outside shoulder width, with the toes pointing forward, the back upright, and the hips and shoulders squarely forward. The weight is distributed equally—50/50—between the right and left sides. The bottoms of both feet are flat to the floor and the knees are bent at a 45 to 90 degree angle, depending on the level of experience, strength, or physical limitations of the practitioner. As with the bo stance, the lower the better for the greatest stability and strength training.

In the horse stance, the body's position is strongest from the side, but not from the front or rear.

Cat Stance

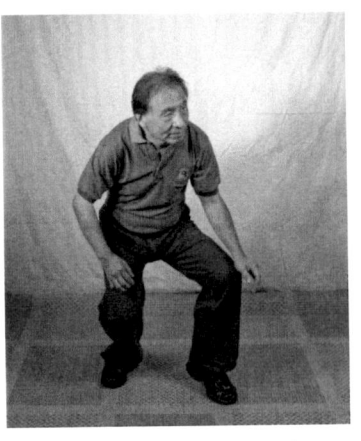

In the cat stance position, one leg is positioned slightly more forward than the rear leg with the front foot contacting the floor with the ball of the foot and the rear foot flat. The distance between the heel of the rear foot and the front foot's instep is about 12 inches for most people. The distribution of weight is about 20 percent on the front leg and 80 percent on the rear leg. The toes of the rear foot point 60 degrees to the side opposite of the front leg, and the front foot's toes point forward. Both knees are bent at a similar degree, with the depth of the stance depending on the level of experience, strength, or physical limitations of the practitioner. Again, the lower the better for the greatest stability and strength training.

Heel Stance

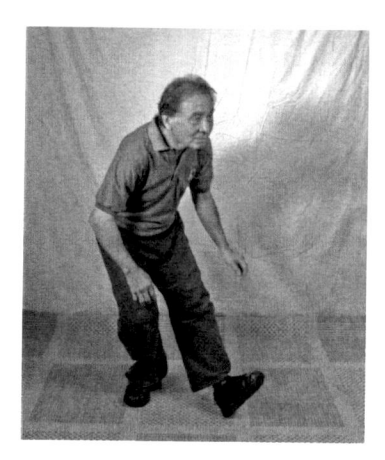

The heel stance is exactly the same as the cat stance except the front foot makes contact with the floor with the heel rather than the ball.

Video

These stances are demonstrated visually in the companion video. Please refer to the Stances section of Individual Postures chapter of the video for more detail.

Stance Exercises

Several of the training exercises in the Breathing chapter of this book are also excellent for improving your stances. Please refer to the Bo, Horse, Cat, and Heel Stance exercises in that chapter for more detail.

DID YOU KNOW?

Stances in martial arts:

The names for the stances used in Lee Family Tai Chi come from Chinese martial arts practice.

The *bo stance* is much like the position an archer would take holding a bow and arrow. It's also sometimes called a "mountain climbing" stance.

The *horse stance* posture is similar to the position of rider or cavalryman mounted on a horse. (For Tai Chi purposes, I prefer to think of it as sitting on a park bench. Much more relaxing!) Both the bo and horse stances help generate power for punches or rooting to prevent being taken off-balance by an opponent.

The *cat stance* is like the fighting posture of the tiger or leopard, animals mimicked in many Shaolin martial arts forms. The position allows for quick, explosive movement, whether it be changing body position, jumping, or launching an attack.

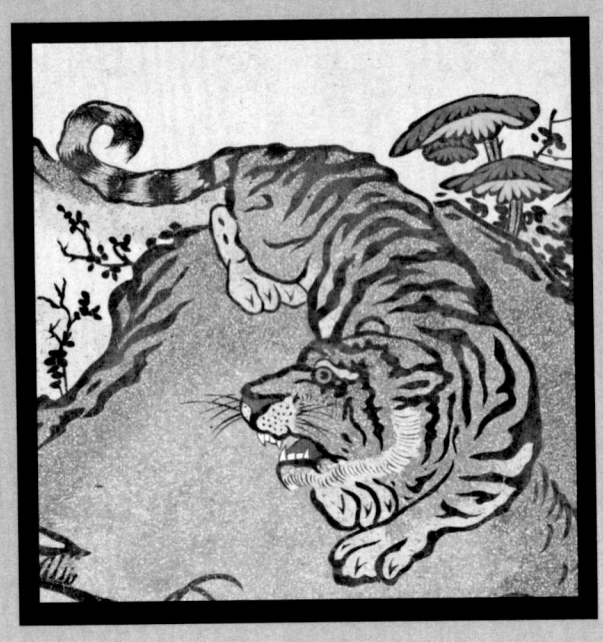

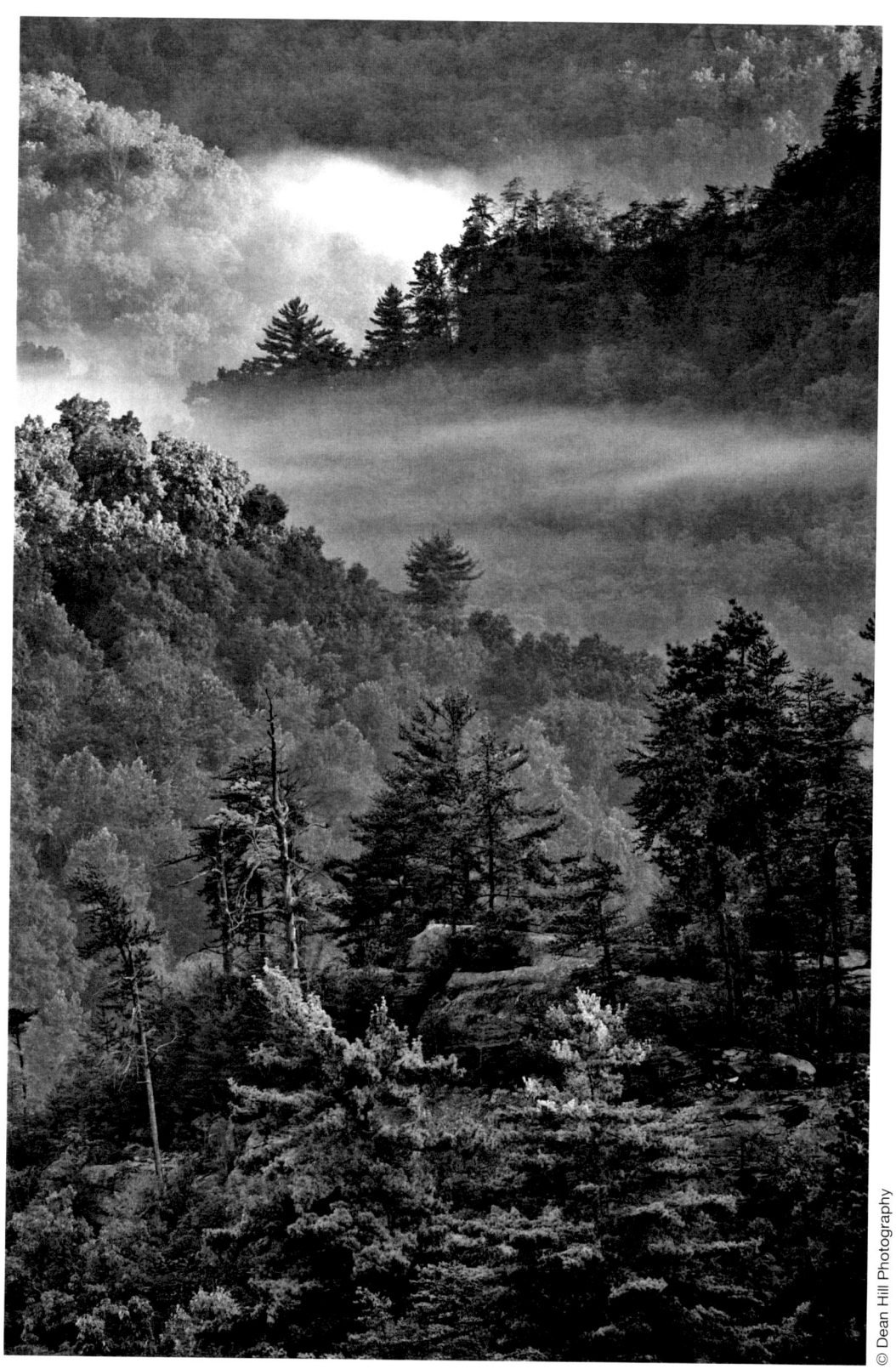

© Dean Hill Photography

128

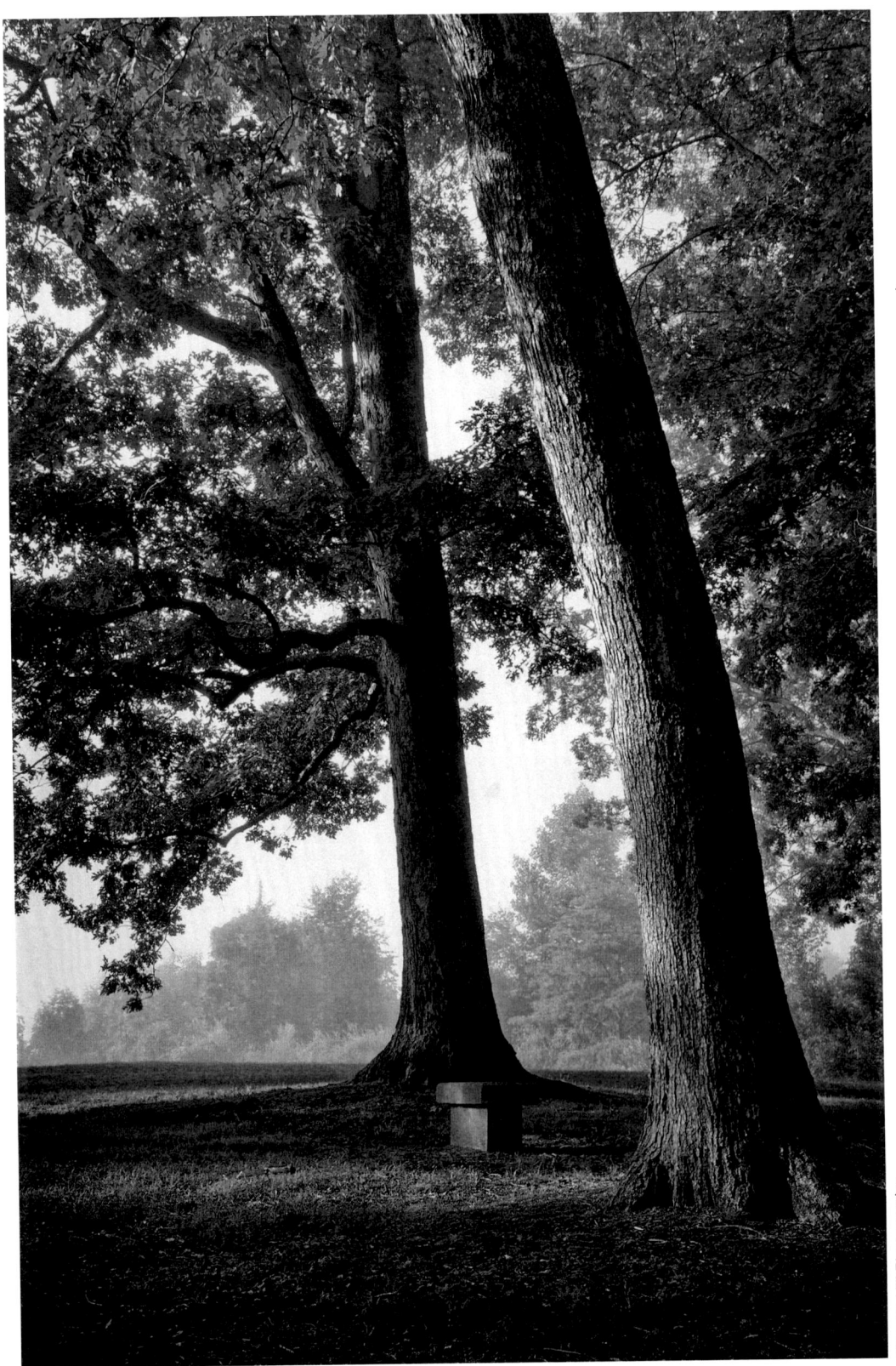

© Dean Hill Photography

EIGHT

WEIGHT TRANSFER & EQUILIBRIUM

WHEN PRACTICING LEE FAMILY TAI CHI, the movements from posture to posture should be done as seamlessly and smoothly as possible, without sudden or jerky movements, as well as without stopping or with long pauses. In Tai Chi, you are constantly in motion, moving from empty to full and back again, soft to strong and back again.

The best way to achieve this unbroken, fluid motion is to be aware of one's equilibrium and transfer of weight from one leg to the other. So what do we mean by equilibrium? The dictionary defines "equilibrium" as: 1) a state in which opposing forces or influences are balanced; 2) a state of physical balance: *I stumbled over a rock but recovered my equilibrium;* 3) a calm state of mind: *His intensity could unsettle his equilibrium.*

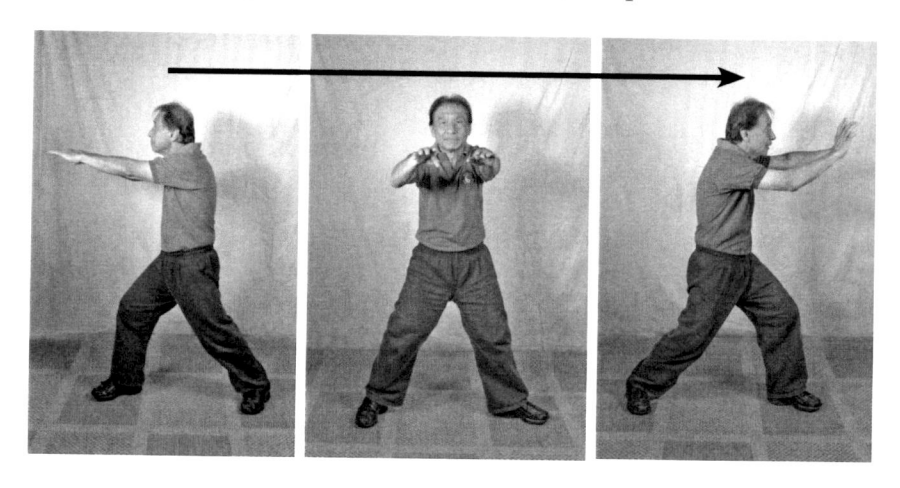

A good example of weight transfer and equilibrium in the Lee Family Tai Chi form is when turning from a right leg forward bo stance to a left leg forward bo stance (postures 17 to 18, for example). At the end of P17, 60 percent of the body's weight is on the front/right leg in a bo stance. Before starting to turn to your left, begin by easing the weight off of your front/right leg, then pivot the right foot on the heel to the left, followed by pivoting the left foot on the heel in the same left direction. You should feel your weight transfer from the right leg to a neutral 50/50 weight position in the middle of the posture, then slowly transfer more weight to the left leg as you bend the left knee and settle into a left leg forward bo stance, facing 180 degrees from where you started. When being conscious of this transfer of weight, you can maintain your equilibrium throughout the posture and move more seamlessly and feel well balanced.

This weight transfer occurs between the inhale and exhale movements within many of the postures and between many of the posture-to-posture transitions. This ability to sense the transfer of weight from side to side, front to back, up to down, etc. helps tremendously with maintaining smooth movement throughout the form, especially on the postures where you are moving to or from being on one leg. Moving lightly and smoothly also helps reduce the stress on the joints of your lower body.

Equilibrium Exercises

Regardless of your stance during the form, it is important for your back to remain perpendicular to the floor to achieve the proper equilibrium. As you transition between moves or raise/step with the foot, you want to achieve a neutral position before you switch your stance. A good way to increase your ability in this area is to practice just a single posture, repeatedly performing the inhale and exhale motions, or repeatedly practice just the transition movement between two postures. The example given above with P17 and P18 can also be done with P21 and P22 to work with turning the other direction.

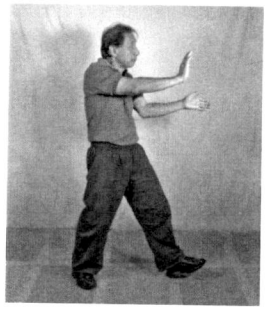

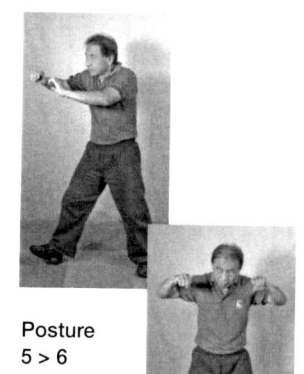

Good drills can also be done with the following movements:

-Posture 2: As the hands lower from overhead, shift the weight to the left leg before raising the right leg. By shifting the weight to the left first, it is much easier to raise the right leg smoothly and with balance. Then step out to a right bo stance to complete the posture. Repeat.

-Postures 13 & 27: This side to side movement can also be practiced with P13, shifting the weight from the 50/50 neutral position horse stance toward the left leg before raising the right leg. Use the mirror image P27 to work with shifting weight from left to right, before raising the left leg.

-Posture 3: Starting in a right side forward bo stance with both arms extended to the front, slowly shift the weight from your right forward leg to your rear left leg. Once your body's weight has shifted from the front leg to the rear leg, then lift your front/right foot off the floor and bring it back to a heel stance. As mentioned above, by shifting weight to the rear first, it is much easier to raise the front leg smoothly and with balance.

-Postures 5, 6, 7 (9, 10, 11): As you turn your body to the left from a 60/40 right foot forward bo stance at the end of P5 to a horse stance in P6, pivot on the heel of the right foot

Weight Transfer & Equilibrium

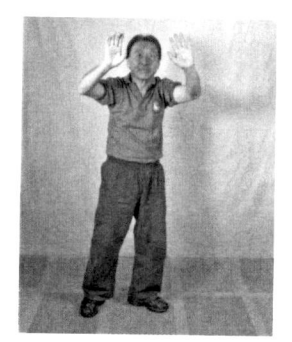

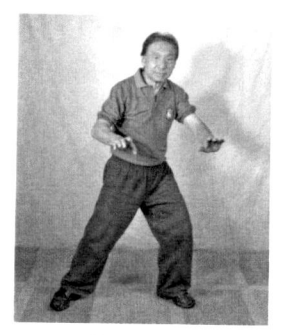

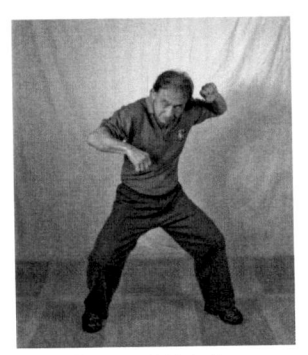

Posture 6 Exhale

first, followed by rotating on the left heel until you are in the 50/50 neutral horse stance. This movement is good for using foot movement to properly transfer your weight.

You can also continue with the exhale portion of P6 body sinking/bending at the knee; as the right fist is directed to the floor. Make sure to bend more by using your quadriceps muscles rather than bending too much at the waist and using your lower back, so that your upper body remains mostly perpendicular to the floor. Then continue with P7, the body rising using your quads, and then the left palm directed towards the floor. This second portion will help develop a greater sense of vertical movement and weight transfer between the upper and lower body.

Perform mirror postures 9, 10, 11 to work with moving from left to right.

Video

This concept of weight transfer and equilibrium is demonstrated visually in the companion video. Please refer to the Transferring Weight and Equilibrium sections of the Individual Postures chapter of the video for more detail.

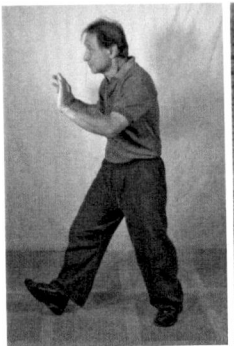

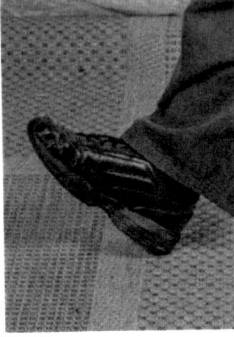

Stepping

One key to making fluid movements and seamless transitions between postures is how you step. I like to call this "Heel/Toe" stepping. When your foot is raised and off of the floor you place the heel of the foot down so that it contacts the floor first, then you roll the foot forward contacting the ball of your foot (the "toe") to the floor. When raising the foot off of the floor, you first lift the heel of the foot off the floor followed by raising the front part of your foot. This method keeps the stepping light and graceful, preventing the more plodding and heavy movements that come from raising and contacting the entire bottom of the foot, heel and ball, to the floor at the same time.

DID YOU KNOW?

Don't Kill the Grass

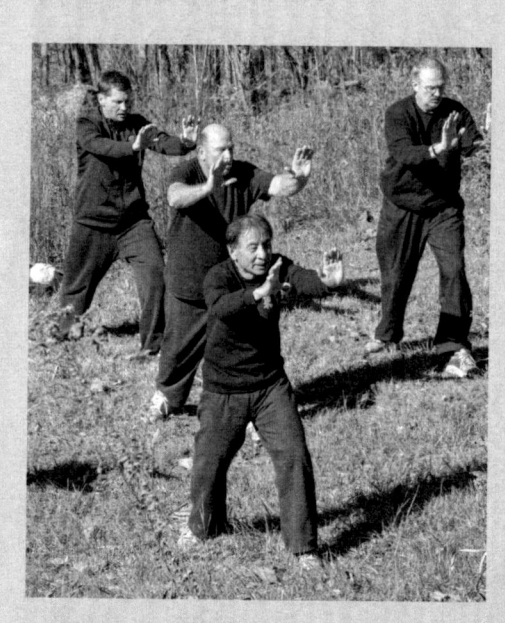

Because we often practiced outdoors on the grass, my grandfather and teacher, Grandmaster Ie Chang Ming, used to tell us not to "kill the grass" when doing Tai Chi. What he meant was for us to make sure we did not drag our feet along the ground, but to raise our feet or move them lightly and gracefully from one posture to the next. As in P3, for example, transferring one's weight first to the rear leg before attempting to raise and bring the front foot back towards the body prevents digging the heel into the ground and dragging it back, "killing the grass." Feel your weight, moving your foot with the body under control.

Weight Transfer & Equilibrium

© Dean Hill Photography

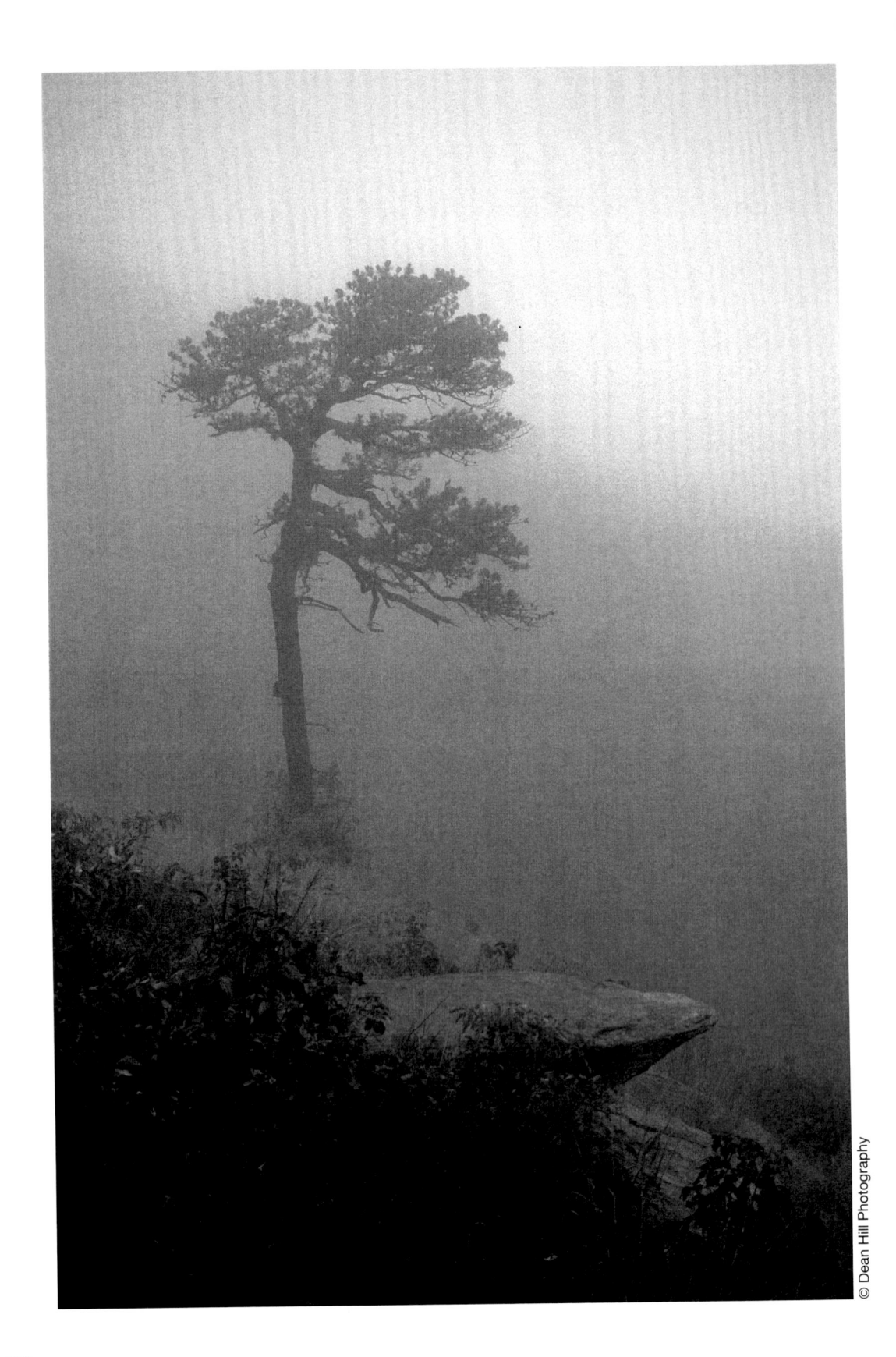

NINE

TARGETING

I've written about making a good connection within yourself throughout this book. The value of gaining this type of awareness and internal feedback is immeasurable for Tai Chi practice and for your overall mental and physical health. One of the best ways to use this ability is with what I call Targeting.

Targeting is using your intent, or Yie, to guide Chi to your vital organs or other areas of the body. We want to use our whole conscious mind to direct this Chi flow so that our vital organs can be as healthy as possible. Targeting can be used to help restore health to poorly functioning organs or to maintain our organ function in an otherwise healthy body.

Targeting is a skill for the more experienced Tai Chi practitioner. It does require greater sensitivity, control and inner awareness, but being new to Tai Chi should not be a roadblock to those who are interested in gaining the benefits of Targeting. I'll include some training tips at the end of this chapter on good ways to work towards Targeting.

The Ten Vital Organs

For the purposes of Targeting, we'll consider ten vital organs, five Yin and five Yang (see Yin and Yang in the

Philosophy chapter). The five Yin organs are the Heart, Lungs, Liver, Spleen, and Kidneys. The Five Yang organs are the Large Intestines, Small Intestines, Stomach, Bladder, and Gall Bladder. I like to work with them as a set of six, using the five Yin organs along with a single grouping of the five Yang organs. I call the Yang grouping the Tan Tien organs or bowels. They are also referred to as "Fu." I like to work with the Main Governing Vessel that runs from the tailbone to the crown of head as an area of focus in Targeting, as well.

Although the organs are connected through the body to the extremities via the meridians (see Philosophy chapter), I don't find it necessary, and it is actually more confusing, to mentally guide your Chi along specific meridians to the organs. When your Chi is circulating naturally, it flows to the areas where it is needed along the proper channels. I like to concentrate on a broader area to target rather than on a bulls-eye or directed there through a precise path. With our intent/Yie and our movements while practicing Tai Chi, we can greatly improve the efficiency and productivity of this circulation.

Personalizing Your Targeting

I like to tell my class that we are all born equal, but we are not born free. By that I mean we all have inherited certain traits and a genetic make-up that can determine much about our health. Some of us may have a family history of heart disease and, even though we jog or do other cardiovascular exercises, could be more susceptible to heart problems because of heredity. The body area I may have as an inherited weakness and need to work on to prevent later problems will be different than yours or others we know.

We can improve this genetic "hand of cards" we are dealt by using Targeting to strengthen those particular organs where we may be weak or that have issues.

Targeting Exercises

So how do we Target? Each of the Tai Chi form's 60 postures is matched to target an organ or set of organs. By practicing the Tai Chi form, Chi will flow to all ten organs and the Governing Meridian by completing the entire set of movements. For the greatest benefit while going through the form, your mind should zoom in on the particular organ that matches that posture. (See appendix A for a list of the organs for each posture. The Form section of this book also has the corresponding organ pictured that matches that particular posture.)

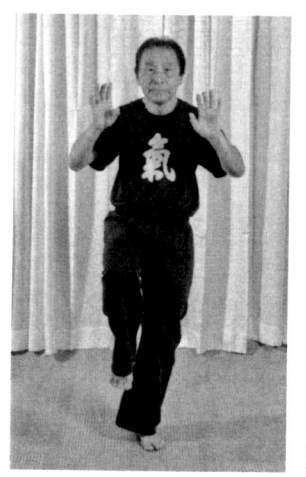

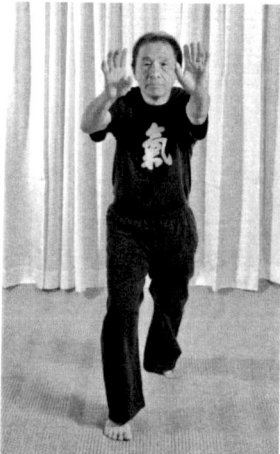

Posture 2-inhale   Posture 2-exhale

As an exercise, let's use Postures 2 and 3 as an example of how to Target:

-Posture 2's matching organ is the lung. When you inhale as you bring your arms down from above and raise your right leg, you also visualize your Chi moving to or gathering in your lungs.

- On the exhale portion of the posture as you step right leg forward into a bo stance and both hands extend out to the front, you visualize your Chi "massaging" or pulsating within the lungs.

-In Posture 3 which targets the heart, move your focus from the lungs to the heart as you shift your weight to the back leg and pull your hands back toward the body on the inhale.

- As you inhale doing the above movement, visualize your Chi moving to or gathering in your heart

Targeting

Posture 3-inhale   Posture 3-exhale

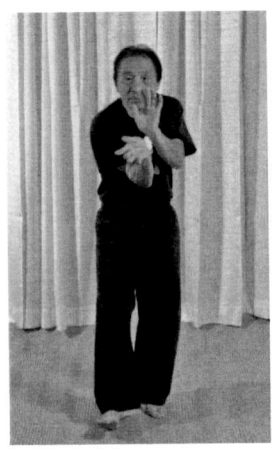

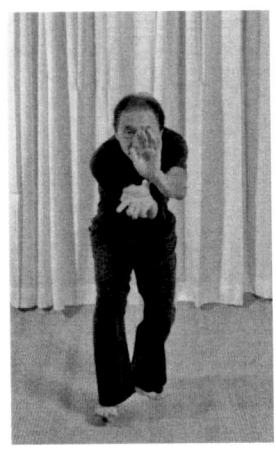

-On the exhale of Posture 3, visualize your Chi "massaging" or pulsating within the heart.

This visualization of gathering and massaging the Chi in the corresponding organ is repeated as you move from posture to posture in the form.

> **PRACTICE TIP**
>
> On the inhale portion of the posture when you first focus your Chi to the chosen organ, you can use your Yie, or intent, to direct the Chi from your Tan Tien to the organ. Although this visualization is not mandatory, many find it helpful since the Tan Tien is an important source of your Chi.

Targeting as you practice the entire form is a great way to globally circulate your Chi throughout your body and to all the organs in a balanced way. If you would like to single out one of two specific organs as I mentioned above, in order to target weak or problem areas, you can also repeat that particular posture on its own or with a set of two or three postures.

Let's first take Postures 6 and 7 as an example. These postures target the intestines (or entire bowel/Yang organs).

- For Posture 6, start from your Horse Stance position with your hands in a light fist beside your head. Inhale fully visualizing your Chi moving to or gathering in your bowel area.

- On the exhale portion of the posture when your right hand moves down toward the floor, visualize your Chi "massaging" or pulsating within the bowels.

Posture 6-inhale   Posture 6-exhale

-Then, in Posture 7, inhale as you raise your stance and your hands open up from the fist next to the head. Maintain your Chi in your bowel area, even directing more Chi there from your Tan Tien.

- As your left palm moves down toward the floor, visualize your Chi "massaging" or pulsating within the bowels.

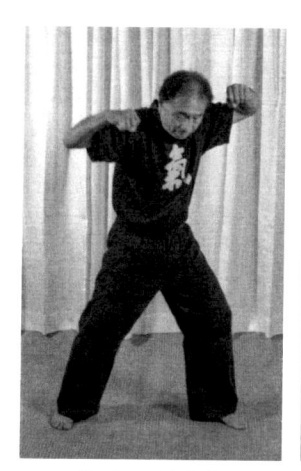

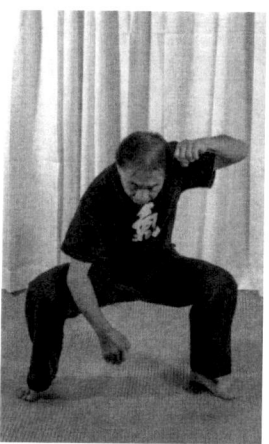

Repeat these movements the desired number of times. Six sets is a good starting point. You can also repeat using Postures 10 and 11, which are the mirror postures to P6 and P7.

> **PRACTICE TIP**
>
> The postures where the wrists are bent at 90 degrees to the arm (P2, P3, P5, etc.) are good for sensing a reflection or rebounding of the Chi that is first directed outward, then back toward the body.

Next, let's take Postures 33 and its mirror 42. These postures target the kidneys. You can also target your lower back/lumbar region.

- For Posture 33, start from your right foot forward Cat Stance position with your hands low and the knees bent. As you rise, inhale fully visualizing your Chi moving to or gathering in your kidneys/lower back.

- On the exhale portion of the posture when your stance sinks and hands move down toward the floor, visualize your Chi "massaging" or pulsating within the kidneys.

Targeting

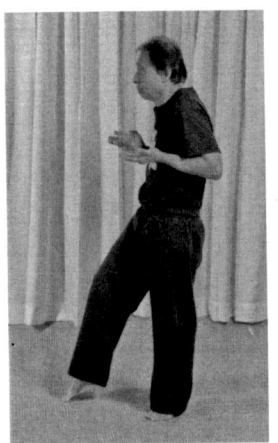

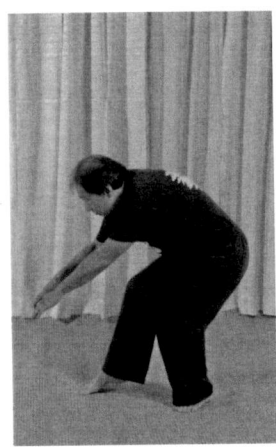

Posture 33-inhale   Posture 33-exhale

Repeat. After six sets, shift to a left foot forward Cat Stance, as in Posture 42, and perform another six sets. I advise you to always do both right foot forward and left foot forward sides of a mirrored posture for a more balanced workout. You can also do the same movements, but place your front foot on the heel rather than the ball part of the foot. This is done Postures in 51 and 57.

These are just three examples of using Targeting with individual Tai Chi postures. You can do this same exercise with any of the 60 postures, or do them in a series of two, three, or more postures as a group. Experiment, and as I always say in my classes, *listen to your own body to tell you what is working well.*

> **PRACTICE TIP**
>
> Your body is good at adapting and can become used to repeating the same posture or movement over time, losing some of its effectiveness with regards to Chi flow and a particular organ. It is a good idea to change up your routine and try different postures, or alternate days performing different types of exercises to keep progress from slowing down.

You can also use some of the single stance breathing exercises described in the Breathing chapter as examples of repeating single postures.

- Opening/Closing Routine: Main Governing Vessel

- Bo Stance Routine: Heart and Lungs

- Horse Stance Routine: Yang Organs/Bowels

- Cat and Heel Stance Routine: Kidneys

Flushing and Flopping

I have used terms like fill, gather, and massage to describe how to think about getting and working with the Chi in the organs. I'd like to discuss two other terms, Flushing and Flopping.

According to traditional Chinese Medicine, many illnesses and injuries are the result of Chi flow that is blocked or restricted in a certain area. Restoring the flow can result in healing. In addition to sensing Chi filling in the organs or pulsating in a massage-like manner, you can also visualize the Chi moving *through* the organ. I call this *Flushing*. You are creating an image of greater motion or flow of Chi that flushes out the organ like clearing out a clogged drain pipe. This flushing also carries out any unwanted toxins or can take the stress off a non-organ area of tension where you may have pain.

Flopping refers to giving a turbocharged boost to your Chi flow. After gathering your Chi in the Tan Tien area by expanding the lower abdominal area on an inhale stroke, you then quickly contract the Tan Tien and push upward with the muscles in that area with a quick and vigorous exhale. At the same time of the contraction, you visualize your Chi rapidly moving up to the targeted area. Imagine energetically squeezing the bottom of a tube of toothpaste, sending the contents out quickly and with greater volume. We often use this technique in our advanced martial arts classes to improve striking power, co-ordinating the flop with a punch. This flopping is equally effective to send a larger amount of Chi to organs or limbs. Be careful not to create too much physical tension or use too much force when flopping, though. With practice, you want to remain relaxed and let the Tan Tien area do the work.

Training Tips For The Beginning Targeter

As I mentioned earlier in this chapter, Targeting does require greater sensitivity, control, and inner awareness. Here are a couple of training tips on how to better develop these skills.

Isolation with the Complete Breath: One of the best ways to help acquire inner body location sensitivity is to practice isolating the three levels of focus of the Complete Breath as detailed in the Breathing Chapter on page 109. To review, the Complete Breath utilizes three levels of focus along the front of the torso—lower, center, and upper. The lower level is your Tan Tien area, the center level is located near the solar plexus, and the upper level is located in the upper lung/chest area. Although these levels do not exactly correspond to any specific organ, they do work with smaller inner areas and the effort to recognize the three distinct levels will help you better isolate and feel smaller areas within your body with more responsiveness and greater command.

The upper level is the easiest level to work with as a beginner, since most people breathe with a focus on the chest. Start with the Complete Breath-Upper Level Only Exercise Two and perform once a day for five minutes each session. If after two weeks or so of practice you feel comfortable with isolating the upper level, move to the center level as described in Exercise Three on page 108. The center level may take a bit more practice to isolate than the other two levels, so a little more time may be required working at the Center Level. Once comfortable with the center level, then work on the Lower Level as described in Exercise One, followed by the All-Level Complete Breath in Exercise Four.

Isolation using the hands: Another method is to work with connecting your consciousness to a particular part of the body via hand contact.

-From a sitting or laying down position, close your eyes and rest the palms of both hands on your chest. Inhale and exhale as before, but on the exhale, intensify your focus on the palms of your hands. As you continue repeating these breathing cycles, try to deepen the focus from your palms into the body and *into* the lungs. Practice for five minutes, then rest.

-From a sitting or laying down position, close your eyes and rest the palm of your right hand on the left side of the chest. Inhale and exhale as before, but on the exhale, intensify your focus on the palm of your hand. As you continue your breathing, try to deepen the focus from your palm into the body and *into* the heart. Practice for five minutes, then rest.

- Repeat as above, placing the palms of the hands on the lower abdomen, focusing on connecting *into* the intestines or bladder.

- Repeat as above, placing the palms of the hands on the lower back over the kidney area, focusing on connecting *into* the kidneys.

- Repeat as above, placing the palm of the left hand on the right side of the torso near the liver, focusing on connecting *into* the liver.

Really Listen and Feel: Almost any attention that you can redirect from the pull of outside stimuli—voice chatter, a whirling fan, car noise— to within yourself, helps to train this inner sensing skill. I encourage you to listen to your heartbeat, really taste your food while chewing, take pleasure in the touch of a loved one. All these methods heighten our inner awareness.

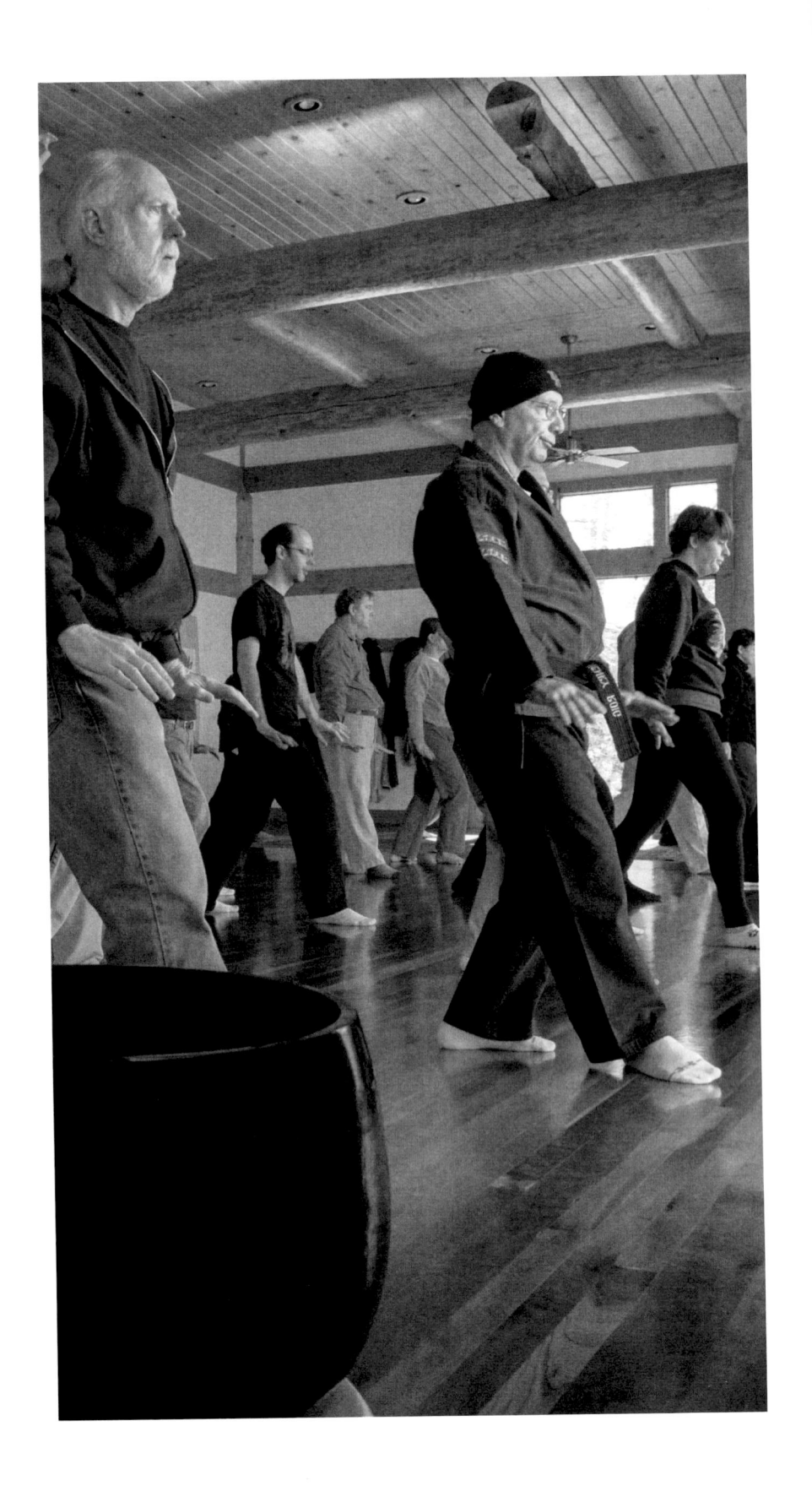

TEN

HOW TO PRACTICE

PEOPLE LEARN IN MANY DIFFERENT WAYS AND AT DIFFERENT RATES OF SPEED. It's no different when learning Lee Family Tai Chi. When we teach the form in person, the beginner level class is one-hour in length and held once a week for a 12-week session. In that time frame, we teach the entire form along with introducing some of the basics about stances, breathing, and give some background.

Most students, though, take the class again, with some people repeating it a number of times. It's not that the form cannot be learned in 12 weeks with diligent practice, but there is so much more to doing Tai Chi than just performing the physical movements. Often, the second time through, more focus can be put on the more subtle details that are discussed—the "whys" and not just the "hows." Correcting postures, gaining greater understanding of stances, balancing, weight transfer, and equilibrium, as well as coordinating the movements with the breathing—all are improved once you gain confidence with the form itself. The impetus for this book and video is to help improve that learning curve.

One of the most important keys to success that I have discovered while observing my students is *persistence*—for them not to grow discouraged. This feeling often happens because they struggle to remember the moves or if they compare themselves to others when it comes to balance, deepness of the stances, or not making any mistakes. Lee Family Tai Chi is not a competitive sport! If you want to use someone else who does the form well as a model or motivation that is *productive*. If you look at someone else and believe you can't do that stance as well or learn it as quickly, then that is *counterproductive*. Stop listening to the competitive mind and focus on putting forth effort. Effort will always produce results.

To my students, I always say that I regret to tell them that there is no "ancient Chinese secret" (like the old TV ad) when it comes to learning Lee Family Tai Chi. The only "secret" is practice, practice, practice—and to give 100 percent effort during that practice. It's no mystery: with Tai Chi, you will get out of it exactly what you put into it.

General Sequence of Learning

Start with learning the complete form. This is much like building the framework of a house. It may seem a bit mechanical at first and not very "meditative," but it establishes the strong foundation needed to eventually make the movements more automatic, with less thought.

Add simple breathing: Since your breathing is such an important component to generating the health benefits of Tai Chi, it is good to add the patterned breathing to the form as soon as possible. Start with simply inhaling and exhaling in sync with movements as described in the book's form section or the video. At this early stage, you can omit focusing on the Tan Tien or other levels. Just simply breathe fully and without straining.

Add Tan Tien Level Breathing: See the Breathing chapter for details of this method. At this next stage, focus is now also on developing your sense of *where* to breathe as you do the form.

Start to examine your stances, weight transfer, and equilibrium: Start paying more attention to these three related concepts as you become more comfortable with doing the form and the breathing. You may want to video yourself doing the form to more closely observe where you are with these areas. Often what we think we are doing and what we actually are doing are two different things.

Don't be too hard on yourself. It is sometimes difficult to look at ourselves performing, but try to be objective and think of the long-term goal of improving your practice. The repetition will also help to develop muscle memory so that the movements become more automatic.

Reduce tension: Overall, make sure you do not become tense. You want to be relaxed, but not limp. You want to have sound, erect posture, but without stiffening the back. You want to sink your stances, but do so without straining. As I tell my classes while they are performing even the most demanding postures, "Don't make faces." A grimace or frown is a sure sign of too much tension.

Add the Complete Breath: Once you have practiced the Three-Level Complete Breath in a standing or sitting position to a point where it has become natural and instinctual, add it to the form. This is the breathing that will generate the most Chi. The Complete Breath is the ultimate level of breathing to do with Lee Family Tai Chi.

Targeting: See the Targeting chapter for details of the method. The form movements and your Tan Tien level breathing should be comfortable at this point before adding targeting of the vital organs.

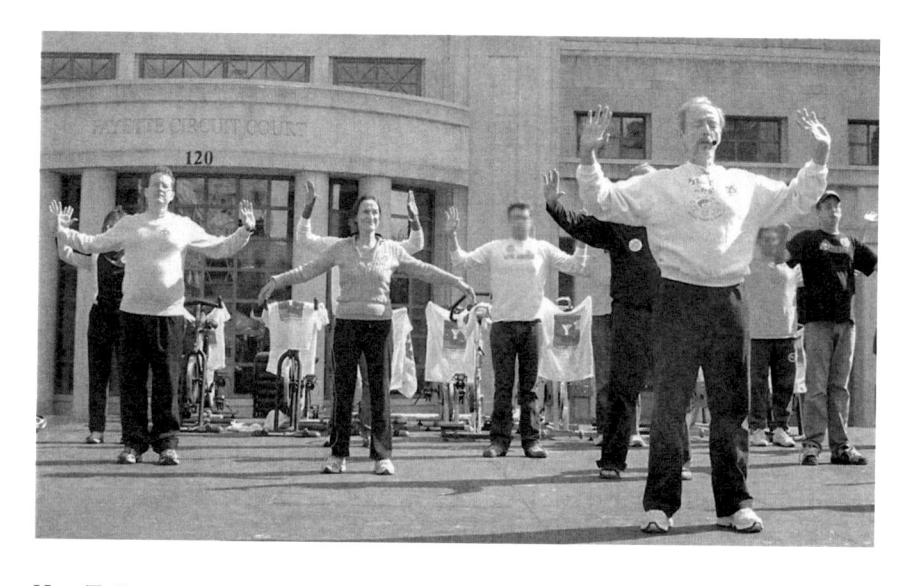

Practice Tips

Practice One Section At A Time: You can also practice and repeat small sections of the form rather than the entire Tai Chi form from beginning to end. This is especially helpful if there is a section that you feel needs extra work in order for you to feel more comfortable, like pivoting smoothly in P4 or turning your stance 180 degrees as with P18, 22, 32, and 41. You can choose just one or two postures to perform and repeat, or put 6-10 postures together depending upon your needs. To help with this, the video divides the complete form into 11 sections of 4-6 postures each.

Flow: When moving from an inhale to an exhale movement, or exhale to inhale movement, you do not come to a complete stop, but the movement is continuous. Think of the end of one posture as actually the beginning of the next posture—there is a slight overlap between the two. Developing this seamless fluidity for the movement in these Chi Kung exercises is very helpful in refining the concept of one continuous movement in the Tai Chi form.

The Circle: One of the advantages Lee Family Tai Chi has is that it does not require a lot of floor space to perform. The practice area is, basically, a circle. The diameter of this circular boundary is about the same as the person's height or about a one-step radius. For example, a six foot man would cover a circular area about six feet in diameter.

Leisure Walk: One good way to describe the form's pace is that it is equivalent to about one-third of the speed of a leisurely walking pace.

Suspended From Above: Maintaining an upright position with the head up is important in many postures. To aid in this feeling, imagine you have a bungee cord attached to the top of your head on one end and to the ceiling above you on the other end. This will help you keep your head up in a relaxed manner and avoid slumping or tilting the head down.

Support Beam: A visualization exercise that helps with balancing on one leg is to imagine you have a sturdy, straight oak beam or pole that runs from your head down thorough the body to the floor. This extra "support" gives a boost to the feeling of steadiness and remaining upright

The Spotter: Another exercise that helps with balancing on one leg is to focus your vision on an vertical object or shape in the room, like a piece of door trim, window sill, or corner. That reinforces the idea of verticality. You can also fix your gaze on a reference spot, like a wall hanging, light switch, or even a lit candle.

Swimming on Land: An excellent metaphor for the feel and pace of doing Tai Chi is the phrase "swimming on land." Imagine that you can breathe underwater and are standing on the bottom of a pool. The water's light resistance to movement would slow your motions, compared to the same actions on land. The amount of force or intent you would use to move fluidly through water mimics the feel you want to achieve on land.

Intent or Yie: The ancient Tai Chi Classics (guides or rules for Tai Chi practice) say, "Use the mind to direct the movements, which will then be light and agile." You use your mind or intent/Yie instead of muscular force to guide actions of the form. Obviously, you are using muscular force to step, turn or move a hand forward, but that signal to move begins in the brain. It is the idea of your intent that is creating the motion. Through repetition and practice while keeping this mindset, you can develop a strong ability to feel as if your body is moving as a result of the commands from your intention. Your Yie is also used for targeting.

Soft/Hard: Another of the "Classics" explains that when one has mastered the techniques of Tai Chi, "one's arms are like iron bars wrapped in cotton." A Tai Chi practitioner is very strong on the inside, but soft and relaxed on the outside. As mentioned above, this is done by reducing any muscular tension or strain when practicing and focusing on the mind-breath and what it is doing on the inside to generate Chi. By shifting one's awareness inward and thinking inside to outside, the inner strength can be better developed and the reduced tension allows for greater Chi flow.

The Furnace: One's energy or Chi is generated in the Tan Tien area like a home's furnace or HVAC system, then circulated outward through the body's "ductwork" to the organs and limbs. Many of the postures in the Tai Chi form use movements whose motions alternate between an inward and outward direction. Visualize the internal movement of your Chi going outward to your organs and limbs, then returning to the Tan Tien area along with those physical motions.

Double The Pleasure: When done at an average pace, the Lee Family Tai Chi form will take around 12 minutes to complete. For an additional benefit, you can repeat the form. Instead of doing posture 60 as you end the form, go from posture 59 directly to posture 2 and repeat the entire form for a longer practice session.

Energy Boost or Calming: Tai Chi practice can provide different results or benefits depending on how you approach your practice. For example, if it is early in the morning and you would like more of an energy boost to start the day, you can deepen some of the stances and breathe with more air volume on each count to generate more work and thereby increase the amount of Chi circulating.

On the opposite end of the spectrum, at the end of a tough, demanding day, it's late, and you would like to clear your mind, reduce stress, and get some sleep, you can go through the form with a different approach. Slow the speed of your physical movement, extend the duration of your breathing a bit, and don't go as low in your stances. You can also focus more on your center level rather than your lower Tan Tien for an even greater calming effect. Be peaceful and let the stress go.

Environment/Outdoors: Your environment plays a big part in achieving good results practicing Tai Chi. Obviously an area with enough space and few distractions is ideal. Better balance can be achieved on a hard, flat surface as opposed to a thickly padded carpet. Outdoors on natural terrain is ideal. Good, quality air is a must since you will be breathing deeply, so avoid areas of strong odors, wearing perfume, or if outdoors, times of high pollution, pollen, mold, and other allergens.

Speaking of being outside, doing Tai Chi in the outdoors can be invigorating. Good Chi is more abundantly available in the potentially oxygen-rich air, from trees, plants and other living things, and even from the earth, stone, sky, and water. Practicing barefoot on the grass or a sandy beach can also be an excellent way to work on improving your lower body's base, creating a stronger foundation.

Tip: Even though a quiet spot is usually desired, use any outside noise or other distractions to your advantage during practice. If one of our goals with Tai Chi is to achieve a state of calmness and be in control of our actions, then the admission of outside forces should have little effect. If a dog barks, child cries, or you hear loud talking, work on accepting the disturbance by concentrating on your breath and continuing to move slowly and intently. You can be aware of the outside distractions—not necessarily blocking them out completely—but use the opportunity to develop the ability to avoid letting them affect you negatively.

Walking: If you like to walk, you can add a form of Targeting by focusing your breath with your steps. Count as you do in the Tai Chi form or standing breathing meditation, timing your steps to sync with your breath.

How To Practice

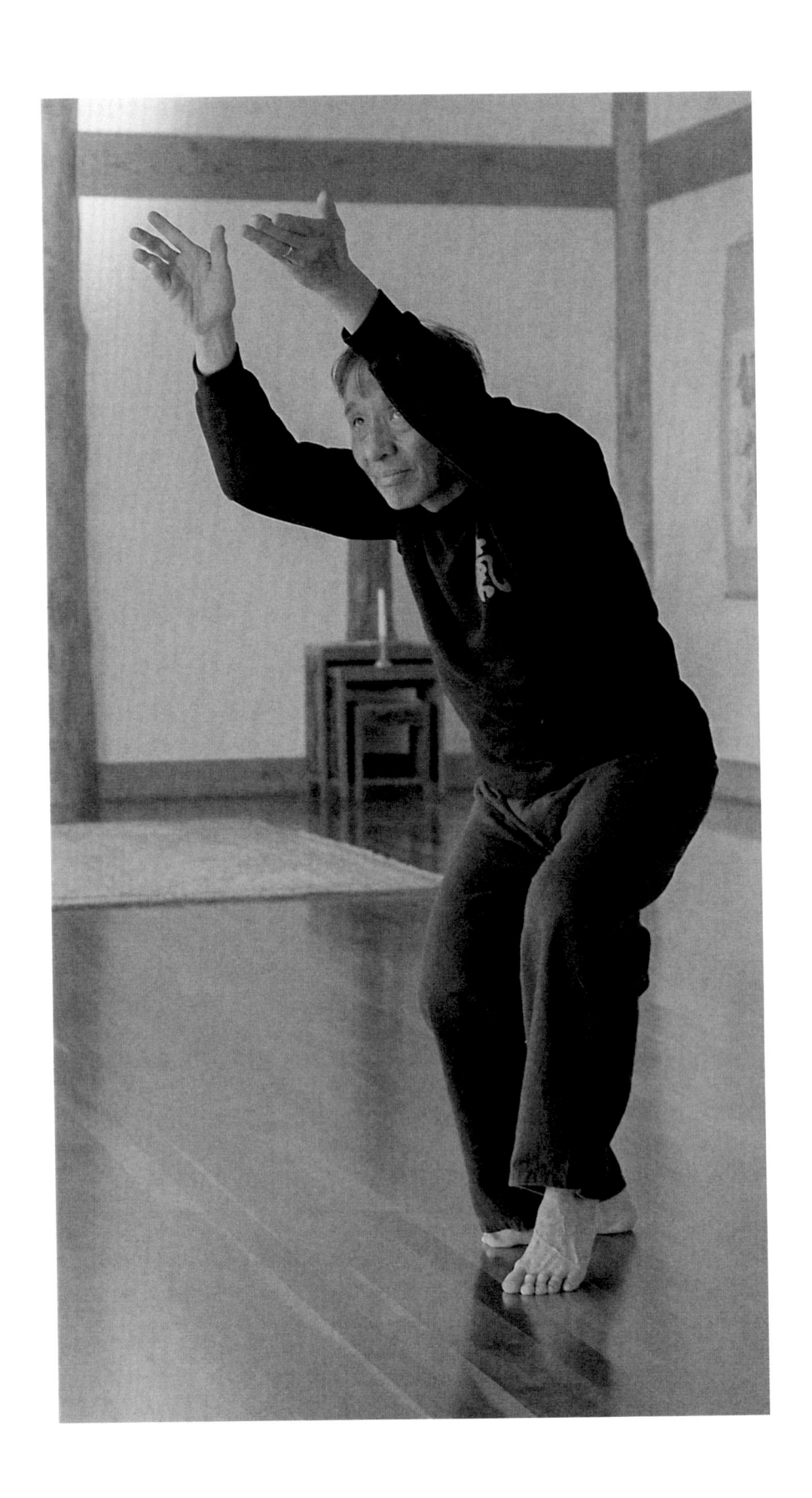

ELEVEN

FREQUENTLY ASKED QUESTIONS

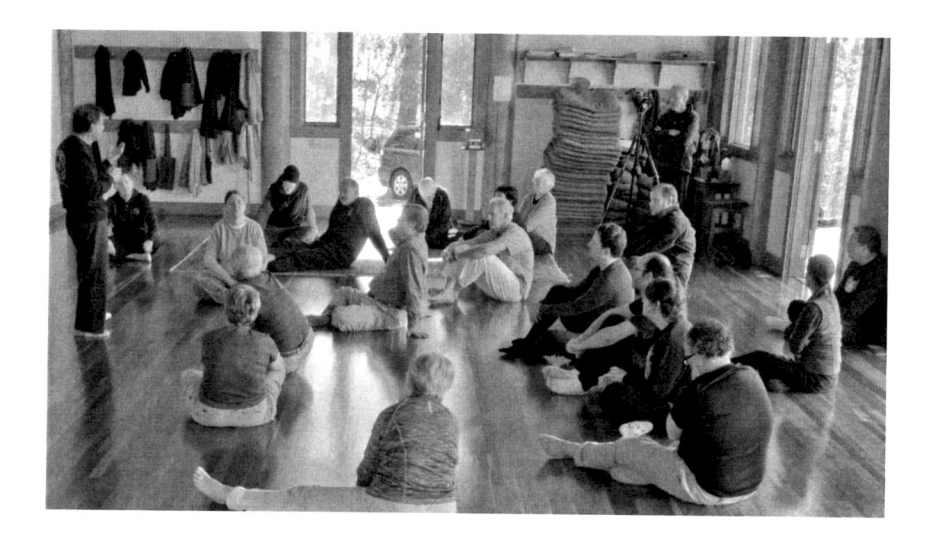

Q: How long does it take to go through the complete form?
A: A 12-minute duration is a good average pace for most people. Beginners can start at around 10 minutes and work their way up. More experienced practitioners can extend to 15-16 minutes. See the Breathing chapter to learn more about setting your pace.

Q: How much should I practice?
A: The more often, the better. I like to say that if you do Tai Chi in the morning, you're not going down that day. Find a way to make Tai Chi practice and meditation part of your daily routine.

Q: Is the time of day important?
A: Any time of day is good, but you can change your approach depending on what you feel you need at that moment. For example, if it's the morning and you'd like to boost your energy for the day, you can be more vigorous by deepening your stances and increasing the time and volume of air. If it is the evening and you'd like to reduce the effects

of a stressful day or aid in sleep, you can slow the pace, reduce the stance depth, and emphasize releasing tension on your exhale motions.

Q: My mind wanders while doing Tai Chi. How can I stay more focused?
A: Counting to yourself while focusing on your breath is not only a good way to set a good, balanced pace, but is a great way to keep your focus on your practice. Targeting your vital organs also holds your attention internally. You can also place a candle in the room or other object to focus on visually while you practice. If your concentration does break, don't become upset or stop your practice. Just bring your awareness back to where you are in the form, to your breath, and to the counting.

Q: Is it better to practice outdoors or indoors?
A: Practicing outdoors can be invigorating. Our natural environment not only has better air to breathe, but the earth, sun, moon, plants, and other living things provide more Chi to absorb. Grass or other natural surfaces also provide good footing to work with your balance. The natural ground also helps disperse your weight, much like a pyramid. If you are indoors, try to find a place that has good air, few distractions, a stable surface, and space to move freely.

Q: How and when did you first learn Lee Family Tai Chi?
A: I learned it from my grandfather and principle martial arts teacher, Ie Chang Ming, while growing up in Indonesia in the early 1960s.

Q: How long have you been teaching Tai Chi and other martial arts?
A: I came to the United States in 1968 to attend the University of Kentucky. While there, I began to teach martial arts. Although I received a Civil Engineering degree, I decided to teach martial arts full-time and have ever since.

Q: Why did you decide to teach Tai Chi to non-martial arts students and is there a difference in how it is taught to the two groups?

A: Lee Family Tai Chi has such wonderful health benefits that I believe it should be available to anyone who is willing to invest their time to learn it. Western science and medicine have finally accepted Tai Chi and other types of meditation as being beneficial, which was not the case when I first began teaching 50 years ago. We use Tai Chi's principles of sensing force and the concept of "soft" and "hard" in our higher level martial arts classes for self-defense training and sparring, but we almost always do LFTC at the end of our two-four hour workouts as a way to recover and re-energize.

Q: What are some of the health benefits of practicing Lee Family Tai Chi?

A: I'm not a doctor, but many of the leading medical and scientific institutions such as Harvard Health, the New England Journal of Medicine, UCLA, and Emory University have published recent research on the benefits of Tai Chi and meditation, including improvements in balance, especially for seniors, core strength, and added flexibility on the physical side. They also cited improvement with mental and emotional issues such as memory, dementia, and depression. Studies have also cited successful treatment of diseases like Parkinson's, diabetes, COPD, and hypertension.

Q: Are there any stories of particular students or practitioners who have been helped by the training that you can share?

A: I had a student walk into her first class with an oxygen tank in tow, then walk out of the last class 12 weeks later without it. One particular student went through multiple rounds of cancer chemotherapy off and on over a 12-year period. She amazed her doctors with her resiliency to keep coming back and regaining her strength to fight another day.

Another, who upon discovering he was suffering from heart disease passed on to him through heredity, was initially told by doctors to avoid anything near strenuous type activity. But after focusing on the internal breathing exercises, along with Tai Chi, he gradually returned to his normal lifestyle and a high level of working out. Those are just three instances out of many, many more that I've experienced.

Q: Can Tai Chi also be used to improve athletic performance?

A: Yes, Tai Chi practice can not only improve the physical attributes of balance, flexibility, and core postural strength that are important in almost every sport or physical activity, but real gains can be made on the mental side, especially with the mind-body connection, heightened awareness, and reducing stress and performance anxiety.

Q: What is "targeting" and how is the health of the internal organs improved with targeting in Tai Chi practice? Is "massaging" the organs similar?

A: Targeting is using your conscious mind to direct Chi to your vital organs or other areas of your body. By guiding more Chi to the organs they can function much more efficiently and can improve problem issues by restoring good circulation where Chi flow may have been restricted. Massaging is how you think about the Chi working or pulsating within the organ when Targeting.

Q: Can you talk some about the concept of "unifying" and making "an internal connection" in Tai Chi practice?

A: The philosophy behind Tai Chi and other meditative exercises is based on harmony or the bringing together of separate elements into balance. The whole is greater than the sum of the parts, if you will. Proper Tai Chi practice combines your body, mind, and spirit. And proper practice is attained by looking inward, listening to your body, paying attention to your breathing, and equally important, by the discipline developed through the effort of focused, frequent practice.

Q: What are meridians and vessels and how do they fit in with Tai Chi practice?
A: Traditional Chinese Medicine lays out the body like a map with a series or rivers, streams, and lakes. But instead of water flow, you have Chi flow and storage along a series of meridians, vessels, and cavities that connect the vital organs through the body to the extremities. Tai Chi practice not only improves the circulation of Chi along this system, but adds the ability to help you control that flow.

Q: Many people are interested in Tai Chi because modern lives have become so over-scheduled, technologically dependent, and stressful. Any advice for people who find it difficult to find the time to practice regularly?
A: Like most things of value, the amount of effort you put into something determines the benefit you derive from it. There are no shortcuts. But I believe that once you start to practice Tai Chi, if you can be determined enough to stick with it until you get that first small taste of the benefits, it will become a healthy habit, something you will *want* to do. The practice time becomes *your* minutes, *your* hours—a time to yourself for recharging and peacefulness that you will look forward to doing each day.

Q: Can Tai Chi be beneficial for senior practitioners who may not be able to perform all of the postures fully?
A: It's definitely a good practice for seniors. Tai Chi is great for improving your balance to protect us from falls, is gentle enough to be easier on the body than many higher impact exercises, and has been found to help slow the aging process. And yes, certain postures can be modified to allow for those with physical limitations. The main adaptation is for postures where you raise up and balance on one leg. You can modify those postures by placing the raised leg so that

the ball of that foot lightly touches the floor next to the other leg. You can also reduce the amount you bend the knees and lower the body on many of the deeper stances. You can also use a chair for support. Set a chair near you and hold on with one hand while moving normally with the other hand. (See appendix B for modification details.)

Q: What would you say are the top three elements in one's practice that can take them to a higher or next level?
A: 1) Practice coordinating your breath with your physical movements in the most seamless, fluid way. Perform the separate breathing and stance exercises, in addition to the form to achieve this.
2) Try to reduce any tension or stress—physical and mental—during the practice. Let all of that go. Be strong on the inside and relaxed on the outside.
3) Always strive to listen to your body and make a good *connection* within yourself. Body/Mind self-awareness.

And one more:
Practice, practice, practice…..then practice some more.

Q: What is the correct pronunciation of your name?
A: Hiang Thè is pronounced "Shung-Tay"

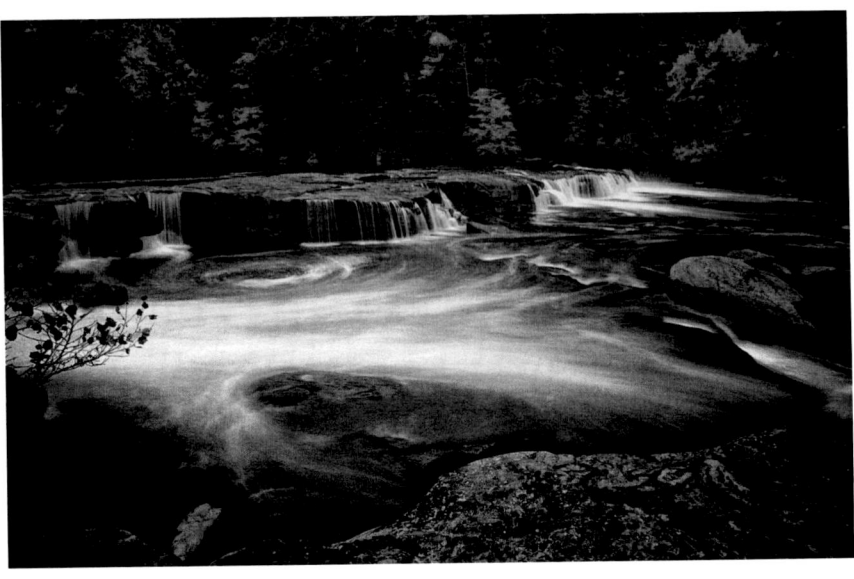

© Dean Hill Photography

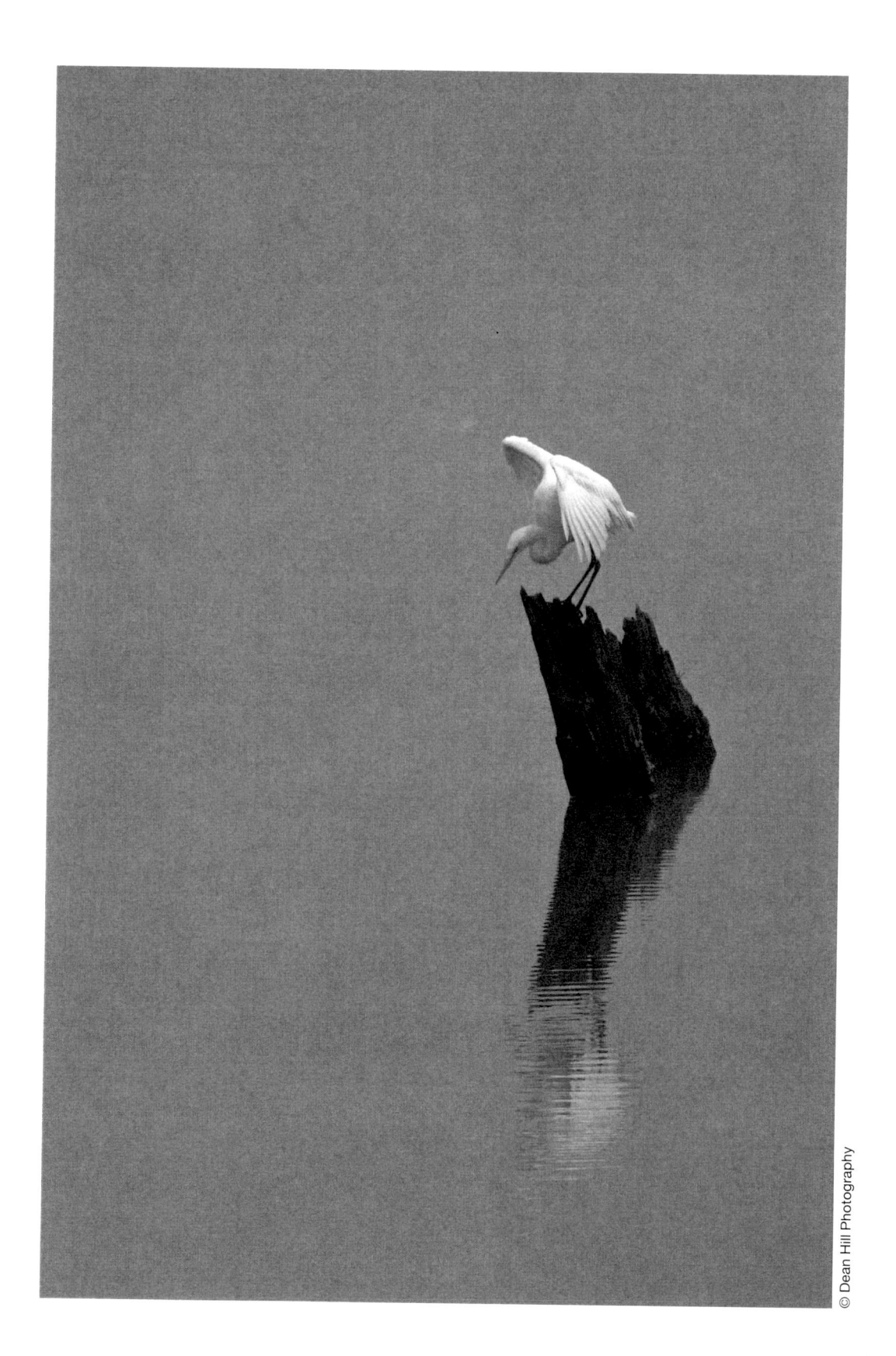

Lung

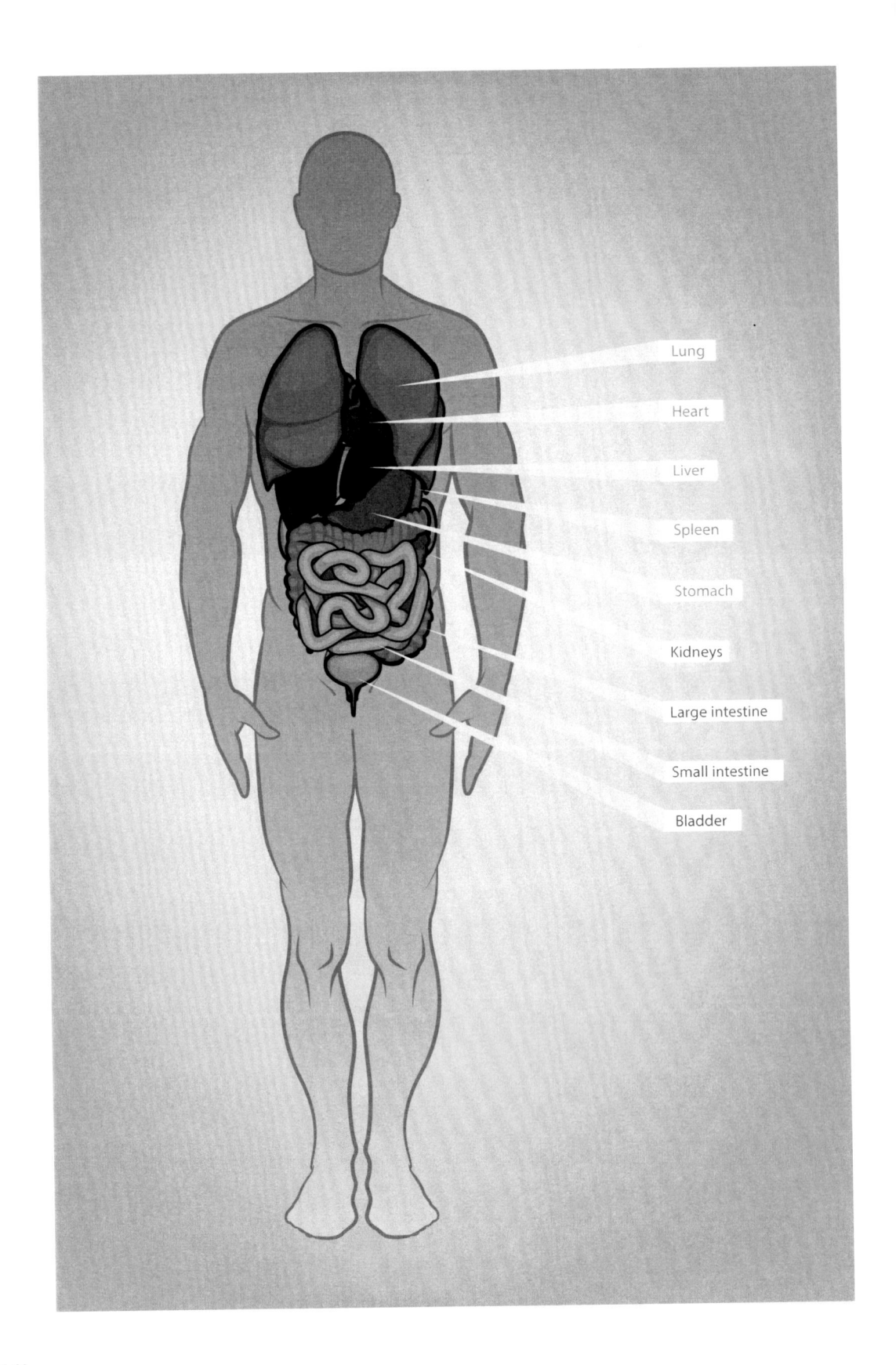

Heart

Liver

Spleen

Stomach

Kidneys

Large intestine

Small intestine

Bladder

APPENDIX A: VITAL ORGANS TARGETED

This list identifies the main vital organ (or the Main Governing Meridian) targeted with each of the form's 60 postures. Other organs can be affected within each posture, especially those physically close to each other such as the heart and the lungs, or the liver and gallbladder, for example.

NOTE: The five Yang organs are small and large intestines, stomach, bladder and gallbladder.

Posture	Targeted Organ
Posture 1	**Main Governing Meridian**
Posture 2	**Lungs**
Posture 3	**Heart**
Posture 4	**Right Lung**
Posture 5	**Right Lung**
Posture 6	**Five Yang Organs**
Posture 7	**Five Yang Organs**
Posture 8	**Left Lung**
Posture 9	**Left Lung**
Posture 10	**Five Yang Organs**
Posture 11	**Five Yang Organs**
Posture 12	**Five Yang Organs**
Posture 13	**Main Governing Meridian**
Posture 14	**Lungs**
Posture 15	**Liver, Kidney, Spleen**

Posture 16	**Heart**
Posture 17	**Lungs**
Posture 18	**Main Governing Meridian**
Posture 19	**Main Governing Meridian**
Posture 20	**Main Governing Meridian**
Posture 21	**Lungs**
Posture 22	**Main Governing Meridian**
Posture 23	**Main Governing Meridian**
Posture 24	**Main Governing Meridian**
Posture 25	**Five Yang Organs**
Posture 26	**Five Yang Organs**
Posture 27	**Main Governing Meridian**
Posture 28	**Lungs**
Posture 29	**Liver, Kidney, Spleen**
Posture 30	**Heart**
Posture 31	**Lungs**
Posture 32	**Main Governing Meridian**
Posture 33	**Liver, Kidney, Spleen**
Posture 34	**Lungs**
Posture 35	**Left Lung**
Posture 36	**Main Governing Meridian**
Posture 37	**Main Governing Meridian**
Posture 38	**Heart**
Posture 39	**Main Governing Meridian**

Posture 40	**Lungs**
Posture 41	**Main Governing Meridian**
Posture 42	**Liver, Kidney, Spleen**
Posture 43	**Lungs**
Posture 44	**Right Lung**
Posture 45	**Main Governing Meridian**
Posture 46	**Main Governing Meridian**
Posture 47	**Heart**
Posture 48	**Main Governing Meridian**
Posture 49	**Lungs**
Posture 50	**Liver, Kidney, Spleen**
Posture 51	**Liver, Kidney, Spleen**
Posture 52	**Lungs**
Posture 53	**Left Lung**
Posture 54	**Main Governing Meridian**
Posture 55	**Main Governing Meridian**
Posture 56	**Liver, Kidney, Spleen**
Posture 57	**Liver, Kidney, Spleen**
Posture 58	**Main Governing Meridian**
Posture 59	**Main Governing Meridian**
Posture 60	**Main Governing Meridian**

APPENDIX B: FORM MODIFICATIONS FOR THOSE WITH PHYSICAL LIMITATIONS

Some people may have physical limitations that prevent them from performing a few of the more demanding postures in Lee Family Tai Chi, but *that should not prevent them from practicing and gaining the benefits of Tai Chi practice.* Below, we have included some modifications to these particular postures that will allow most people to still practice the complete form. For some, these adjustments will make good step-by-step training towards gradually achieving the full movements over time.

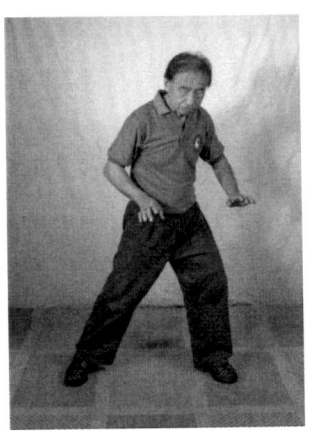

Postures 13/14 & 27/28

For the inhale portion of Posture 13, instead of completely raising the right foot off the floor, keep the front part of the foot in light contact with the floor as you bring it in toward the left foot. Do the same with your left side on Posture 27.

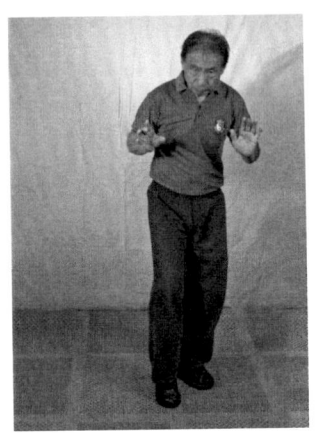

For the exhale portion Posture 13, instead of extending the right leg out parallel to the floor, raise the right foot (or slide it forward) and place it down in front of the body, lightly tapping the ball of the foot onto the floor while still keeping most of your weight on the back/left leg. Do the same with your left side on Posture 27.

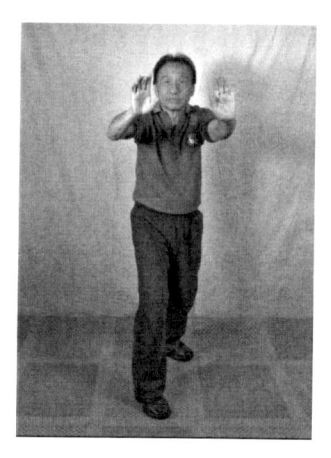

For the inhale portion of Posture 14, bring the right foot back next to the left foot, but keep it in contact with the floor as you do so. Step out to a right bo stance as normal for the exhale portion. Do the same with your left leg on Posture 28.

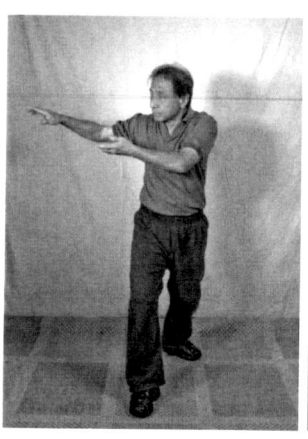

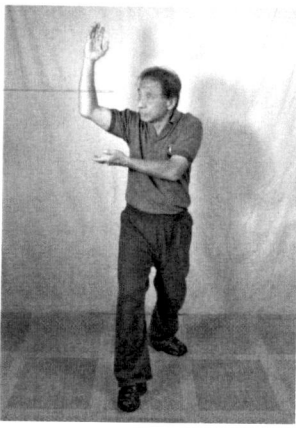

Postures 15 & 29

For the inhale portion of Posture 15, instead of completely pivoting the body to the right, keep your stance facing forward, but move just your arms and upper body to the left as you turn at the waist. Do the same with your left side on Posture 29.

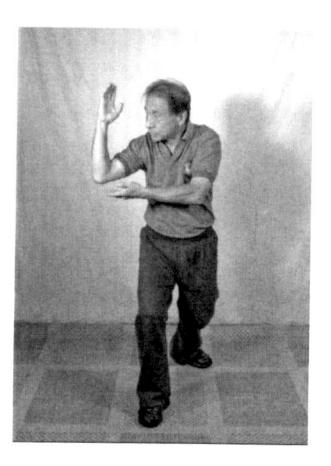

For the exhale portion of Posture 15, keep your stance facing forward and bend the right knee to sink your stance. Do the same with your left side on Posture 29.

Appendix B

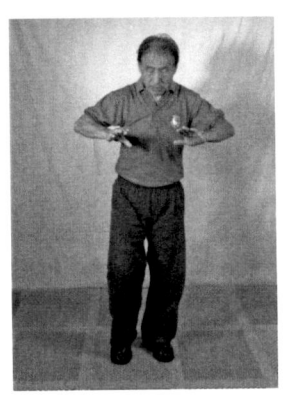

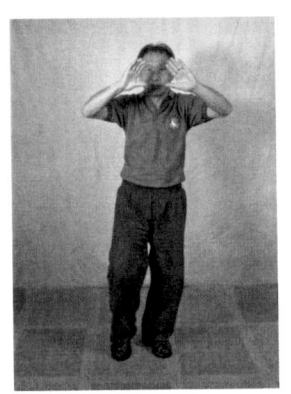

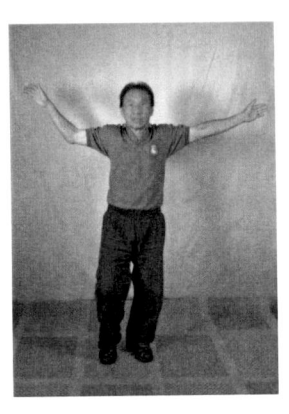

Postures 19/20 & 23/24

For the inhale portion of Posture 19, instead of completely raising the right foot off the floor, keep the front part of the foot in light contact with the floor as you bring it in beside the left foot. Arms raise as normal. Do the same with your left side on Posture 23.

For the exhale portion of Posture 19, keep the front part of the right foot in light contact with the floor as your arms lower out to the sides. Do the same with your left side on Posture 23.

Keep the right foot in contact with the floor on the inhale portion of Posture 20, then that foot rests completely flat as you finish the exhale portion. Do the same with your left side on Posture 24.

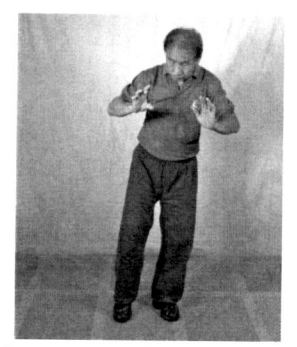

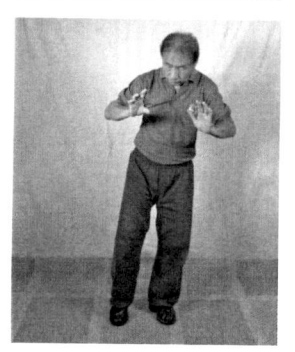

Postures 39/40 & 48/49

For the inhale portion of Posture 39, instead of completely raising the right foot off the floor, keep the front part of the foot in light contact with the floor as you bring it in beside the left foot. Arms raise to the front of the chest as normal. Do the same with your left foot on Posture 48.

For the exhale portion of Posture 39, keep the front part of the right foot in light contact with the floor as you slide it out to the right side. Bend the left knee and lean the upper body to the left if possible. Do the same with your left leg on Posture 48.

For the inhale portion of Posture 40, slide the right foot back next to the left foot as your upper body moves to an erect posture. Do the same for the inhale portion of Posture 49, sliding the left foot back next to the right foot.

Using A Chair

A chair can also be used to help work with your balance.

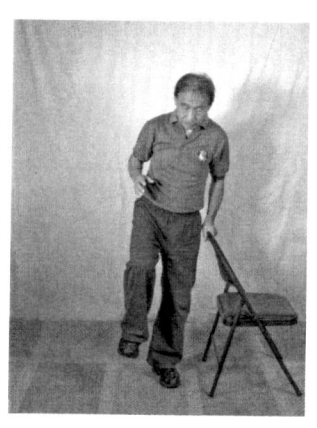

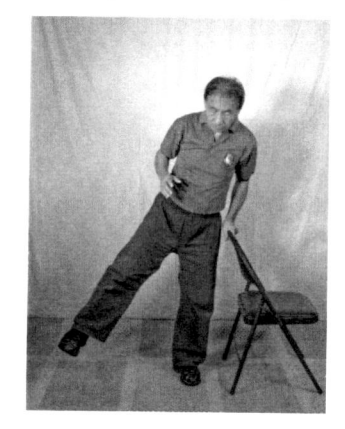

Place one hand on a nearby chair while either practicing the complete form or individual postures.

Appendix B